Improving Animal Welfare: A Practical Approach

Improving Animal Welfare:
A Practical Approach

Edited by **Ryan Webber**

□ SYRAWOOD
PUBLISHING HOUSE

New York

Published by Syrawood Publishing House,
750 Third Avenue, 9th Floor,
New York, NY 10017, USA
www.syrawoodpublishinghouse.com

Improving Animal Welfare: A Practical Approach
Edited by Ryan Webber

© 2016 Syrawood Publishing House

International Standard Book Number: 978-1-68286-010-6 (Hardback)

Printed in the United States of America.

Contents

Preface

Animal welfare plays a crucial role in agricultural practices like animal husbandry and dairy farming. This book is a compilation of chapters that discuss the most vital concepts and emerging trends in the field of animal welfare. Various aspects of animal behavior, physiology, reproduction, etc. have been discussed in a lucid manner. The book is appropriate for students of veterinary sciences, zoology and similar disciplines seeking detailed information, as well as for professionals engaged in this field, as it includes contributions of experts and scientists which will provide innovative insights into this subject.

The information shared in this book is based on empirical researches made by veterans in this field of study. The elaborative information provided in this book will help the readers further their scope of knowledge leading to advancements in this field.

Finally, I would like to thank my fellow researchers who gave constructive feedback and my family members who supported me at every step of my research.

Editor

Effectiveness of Gel Repellents on Feral Pigeons

Birte Stock * and Daniel Haag-Wackernagel

Department of Biomedicine, University of Basel, Pestalozzistrasse 20, 4056 Basel, Switzerland;
E-Mail: daniel.haag@unibas.ch

* Author to whom correspondence should be addressed; E-Mail: birte.stock@unibas.ch.

Simple Summary: Feral pigeons live in close association in urban areas. They constitute serious health risks to humans and also lead to high economic loss due to costly damage to buildings, historic monuments, statues and even vegetation. While numerous avian repellent systems are regularly introduced onto the market, scientific proof of efficacy and their use from the point of view of animal welfare is lacking. Therefore, two avian gel repellents were studied on free-living feral pigeons in this study. The focus was set on repellent efficacy and animal welfare concerns. This study's aim is to contribute to a better understanding of feral pigeon management in our cities.

Abstract: Millions of feral pigeons (*Columba livia*) live in close association with the human population in our cities. They pose serious health risks to humans and lead to high economic loss due to damage caused to buildings. Consequently, house owners and city authorities are not willing to allow pigeons on their buildings. While various avian repellents are regularly introduced onto the market, scientific proof of efficacy is lacking. This study aimed at testing the effectiveness of two avian gel repellents and additionally examined their application from animal welfare standpoint. The gels used an alleged tactile or visual aversion of the birds, reinforced by additional sensory cues. We mounted experimental shelves with the installed repellents in a pigeon loft and observed the behavior of free-living feral pigeons towards the systems. Both gels showed a restricted, transient repellent effect, but failed to prove the claimed complete effectiveness. Additionally, the gels' adhesive effect remains doubtful in view of animal welfare because gluing of plumage presents a risk to feral pigeons and also to other non-target birds. This study infers that both gels lack the promised complete efficacy, conflict with animal welfare concerns and are therefore not suitable for feral pigeon management in urban areas.

Keywords: capsaicin; *Columba livia*; contact gel; feral pigeon; optical gel; repellent gel

1. Introduction

The feral pigeon, the descendant of the domesticated form of the wild living Rock Dove (*Columba livia*), is a highly successful urbanophilic species, which occurs worldwide. With a domestication history of several thousand years [1], feral pigeons are well adapted to human environments. Due to the abundant feeding options in our cities, feral pigeons have expanded their originally granivorous diet to an omnivorous one [2]. In addition to the positive nutritional effects, cities with house facades, churches and statues offer an ideal environment for the birds. Pigeons that originally lived along coasts with cliffs now use numerous structures associated with urban buildings as roosting, resting, nesting and outlook spots. The close association of large feral pigeon populations and humans creates a human-wildlife conflict with serious health risks. With more than 100 human pathogenic microorganisms and 18 ectoparasites associated with feral pigeons [3,4], the epidemiological significance of these birds to humans is evident. Although the risk of zoonotic diseases caused by feral pigeons is rare, fatal cases have been reported [5]. Besides the medical risk, feral pigeons living in urban habitats also lead to high economic loss due to significant damage to buildings, historic monuments, statues and even vegetation [2]. The removal of pigeon droppings from buildings causes high costs [6]. With an individual pigeon producing around 4–11 kg of excrement each year [7], enormous quantities of pigeon droppings end up in every larger city of the world. This excrement offers a substrate for the growth of microorganisms that are able to destroy building materials [8].

In addition to these negative esthetic and hygienic aspects, the costs of feral pigeons living in urban environments are high. The estimated damages per feral pigeon per year including pollution of buildings, streets and places, as well as hygienic costs, agricultural costs and bird strikes range from 23.7€ to 33.5€ [9], which equals approximately $US 31 to 44. In the USA, the damage caused by feral pigeons has been estimated to $US 1.1 billion per year, not including environmental damage associated with the pigeons serving as reservoirs and vectors for diseases [10]. The relevance of pigeons is further pointed out by the number of about 22'500'000 hits when entering the words "pigeon problems" into the internet search engine Google (accessed 28 October 2013).

Frequently recommended solutions to solve the pigeon problems in residential areas and city centers include a large number of nonlethal systems that repel and exclude the birds from buildings and monuments. Repellents can be used to manipulate animal behavior in a way that an animal is motivated to avoid the consequences of the aversive signal [11]. In general, animal repellent systems can be of visual, acoustic, tactile, olfactory, or gustatory nature, or even combine several of these characteristics [11–17]. The business of production and installation of avian repellent systems involves the sales of millions of dollars worth of products in Europe and the USA [9,18,19]. While netting and other exclusion systems are successfully used against pigeons, these methods do not always seem to be an economic or practical option [20], and such eye-catching systems often distract from the architectural impression [21]. In particular, historic buildings are sensitive to pigeon droppings and difficult to protect from these birds. With the sheltered niches, crevices and ledges common to ornamental facades, such buildings offer ideal nesting and roosting habitats [22]. Several other proofing products promise an optimal integration in the esthetic impression of building facades since they are inconspicuously and discretely mounted onto the affected structure or area. Whereas for example netting and spikes repel the pigeons on the basis of exclusion via mechanical barriers, other innovative systems are often supposed to work with aversive cues that motivate the bird to avoid the treated spaces. These new systems, which are regularly introduced onto the market, promise to be the ideal solution to the problems caused by pigeons on buildings. They are supposed to be not only effective, but also inconspicuous, easy to mount and available at a competitive price. However, data to support the expected results of these new, inventive and allegedly persistently effective bird repellents is rare or inexistent. Furthermore, these new products have rarely been put to test under the point of view of animal welfare. Given the fact that highly motivated pigeons are able to overcome almost every system [19], the effectiveness of new bird repellent products should be investigated critically.

A reasonable feral pigeon management in urban areas requires very good knowledge of proofing and scaring systems and the reactions of the birds towards them. We therefore tested two nonlethal, food-grade, avian repellent gels that are supposed to combine an easy and discrete installation with 100% success in removing the birds from treated areas within less than a week. While one gel is based on the alleged tactile aversion of the birds to capsaicin, the other claims to function through a visual repellent effect that is reinforced by ingredients that are repulsive to the olfactory, gustatory and tactile senses of the birds.

The objective of our study was to assess the effectiveness of these two avian gel repellents by analyzing the behavior of feral pigeons when confronted with them. In addition to the efficacy of the products, we also focused on the gels from the point of view of animal welfare.

2. Materials and Methods

2.1. Study Area

We conducted our study in the pigeon loft of the St. Matthew Church, which is situated in a residential district of Basel, Switzerland (47.5671°N, 7.5930°E). The city of Basel is located in northwestern Switzerland, at the intersection of Switzerland, Germany and France. In August 2012 it counted around 170'000 inhabitants. The climate is continental and during the study period, average temperatures ranged from 20.7 °C in August to 10.7 °C in October.

The pigeon loft was situated above the nave of the church at a height of about 18 m above ground. Besides a floor space of 28 m^2, the loft had 39 nesting boxes and several roosting bars. We set a timer for constant diurnal rhythm of 9 hours and 30 minutes of light and 14 hours and 30 minutes of dark in the loft. The experiments were performed under natural conditions without offering any food or water. The pigeons used the loft exclusively for roosting and breeding. Their food was generally foraged in the surrounding area and the city [23].

2.2. Tested Bird Repellent Gels

Two avian repellent gels were tested on free-ranging feral pigeons: a contact gel and an optical gel. Both products are used in pest bird management programs to protect structures from birds. Since repellent products are continuously changing their names or reentering the market only slightly modified, we refrain from providing the names of the products and the manufacturers. Instead, the tested products stand for a specific but conventionally used kind of repellent system.

2.2.1. Contact Gel

As specified by the manufacturer, the contact gel included non-toxic, 100% natural ingredients and can be used to protect all kinds of indoor and outdoor surfaces of buildings, monuments and also statues against nuisance birds, especially pigeons. The gel contained 0.0357% capsaicin, which is the pungent element of red pepper [24]. According to the distributor, capsaicin causes a mild harmless irritation when being transferred onto the feet of the birds by landing on the treated areas. This sensory reaction to the gel is supposed to condition the pigeons to avoid the location. The clear, odorless and semi-solid gel was supplied in 300 mL cartridges and applied on the experimental shelves in a wave pattern at a stretch according to the application instructions. The distributor claimed that 100% of the bird population would be successfully removed within seven days of gel application, which was allegedly proven during rigorous testing carried out by the developers.

2.2.2. Optical Gel

The second bird repellent, which was examined, was an optical gel, sold by another distributor. According to the general product information, the gel is patented and contains food-grade natural oils. It is supposed to repel all birds from all indoor and outdoor structures without causing any harm to target animals. Ingredients in the product include polyisobutylene, grease lubrication, peppermint oil and cinnamon oil. According to the distributor, the gel is able to repel the pigeons visually because it is perceived as fire within the ultraviolet visual range of the birds. Furthermore, the distributor claimed that natural oils, which should be abhorrent to a bird's senses of smell, taste and touch, reinforce the visual repellent effect. The gel was delivered in 250 mL cartridges with supplementary application dishes of 7 cm in diameter. We applied 15 g of the repellent gel in each dish as recommended in the manufacturer's guidelines.

After consultation with the distributor who determined the number and location of dishes on the experimental shelves, we arranged eight dishes per shelf in two parallel rows of four dishes. The dishes covered a total of 17% of the shelves. The greatest distance between two dishes was 13 cm. According to the application guide, this distance referred to an area with high bird density. The manufacturer claimed that after two or three days even the most dominant birds would avoid the treated areas.

2.3. Study Animals

The feral pigeon colony used for this study contained about 85 birds with an average body weight of 322 g. Due to the fact that the pigeon loft was freely accessible to every feral pigeon in the surrounding area and the birds of our study were able to enter and leave the loft at will, fluctuation of the population was possible. We routinely caught, ringed and weighed the resident pigeons every six months. During the study period, one pigeon that hatched in the loft became integrated into the population, another adult pigeon immigrated and six pigeons, both adults and young, left the population. Due to the periodical flock controls and the cleaning of the pigeon loft twice a month, the pigeons were habituated to human presence. Even though all pigeons of the loft were ringed, either directly as nestlings or as immigrated adults, the small ring numbers were not recognizable on the video material. An unambiguous assignment of the observed reactions of the pigeons to a particular bird was thus not performed.

2.4. Experimental Design and Data Collection

We installed four experimental shelves of 0.6 m length and 0.3 m width as resting, roosting and outlook spots for the pigeons in the loft. Each shelf was attached onto the wall at right angles, offering the birds a convenient area to perch. The shelves were placed in a zigzag pattern at heights of 0.8 m to 1.6 m, about 1.3 m away from the nesting boxes on the adjacent wall. After the installation, the pigeons were given ten days to get used to the new structures in the loft. We performed our experiment in August–October 2012. It consisted of two main phases: a pretrial of 16 days and a trial phase of 26 days. We monitored the experiment with a video camera (JVC model GY-HM150E, Yokohama, Japan) at random dates each for 24 hours. On 27 August 2012, we started the pretrial phase during which we video recorded three out of 16 days in a weekly rhythm to get a base value for the daily use of the shelves without the installed repellents. The dishes in which the optical gel was applied were not mounted during the pretrial phase. The idea was to first create a natural scene with an ordinary structure frequently used by pigeons and not treated with any kind of repellent or uncommon system. Each of the gels was applied on two of the experimental surfaces, according to the distributor's guidelines, on 12 September 2012. However, the shelves and the wall on to which they were installed were thoroughly cleaned before application, as the products are said to only have full effectiveness when used on unsoiled structures, free from any bird excreta. We recorded 16 days of our 26 days trial phase, with the last recorded day being trial day 26. Due to methodological considerations, we eliminated the first trial day of the visual gel testing and restarted the experiment on the second day of recording. As a result, we excluded the first trial day from statistical analyses and assigned the actual second trial day as the first. Thus, the last recorded day of the visual gel testing was trial day 25.

In addition, the emissions and the lifetime of the excited states of the optical gel was measured as it is supposed to be perceived as fire within the ultraviolet visual range of the feral pigeons. The measurements were taken with the compact fluorescence lifetime spectrometer Quantaurus-Tau C11367-11 by Hamamatsu excited at a wavelength of 280 nm.

2.5. Animal Welfare Point of View

We conducted the experiments with the animal experimental permission of the Cantonal Veterinary Office of Basel-Town, Switzerland (authorization No. 2296). The study conformed to Swiss law on animal welfare. The permission allows experiments on animals causing mild stress, which corresponds to the severity Grade 1. According to Swiss animal welfare, severity Grade 1 studies include interventions and manipulations on animals for experimental purposes, which subject the animals to a brief episode of mild stress (pain or injury). Furthermore, it is claimed in Article 4(2) of the Swiss Animal Welfare Act that no person may, without justification, inflict pain, suffering, or injury upon an animal or cause it fear, or disregard the dignity of the animal in any other way. With this in mind, we first tested the pigeons' behavior towards the gels applied in nesting boxes during a test run. During this test run, the pigeons entered their nesting boxes in all cases. Apparently, the birds were not repelled by the gels due to their high motivation to repossess their breeding places. Furthermore, because the chances of nestlings and inexperienced juvenile birds getting into contact with the sticky gels were too high, the nesting boxes test run was canceled prematurely. For that reason we chose to test the repellent gels on new, rather unpopular, experimental shelves in heights starting at 0.8 m so that nestlings and badly flying juveniles were not able to smear the sticky products into their not yet fully grown plumage. With these low motivation structures, not being as fiercely contested as other areas in the loft, the risk of gluing of plumage of adult pigeons was further minimized.

2.6. Data Analysis

We evaluated the recorded behavior and analyzed the number of approaches and landings, as well as the time spent on the experimental shelves prepared with the two repellents for each recorded day. A successful repellent system reduces the number of birds using the protected structure by 100%. Although a general reduction might seem effective to non-experts, only a complete protection marks a successful repellent system. Even low numbers of pigeons still using and soiling the treated areas point out the failure of the repellent system. For the simple reason that even a single pigeon is able to transmit human pathogenic diseases, a repellent system should not only reduce the number of pigeons using a treated structure, but completely remove the birds from it. Due to this reason, the success of the repellents was determined as a reduction of feral pigeons' use of the experimental shelves by not less than 100%.

Based on the claim of the contact gel distributor, complete avoidance of the prepared shelves was to be expected within seven days of gel application. We therefore categorized three trial phases: pretrial (three recorded days), trial Days 1–7 (five recorded days) when full effectiveness was not yet expected and trial Days 8–26 (11 recorded days) when complete effectiveness was anticipated.

For the visual gel we similarly analyzed the number of approaches and landings, together with the time spent on the shelves. The distributor of the visual gel claimed that the product would be absolutely effective within three days of product application. We characterized three trial phases: pretrial (three recorded days), trial Days 1–3 (two recorded days) and trial Days 4–25 (13 recorded days). Additionally, we distinguished between different behaviors of the pigeon towards the visual repellent: (a) approach without landing and therefore no possible contact, (b) landing with immediate gel contact, (c) subsequent gel contact, and (d) no contact with the gel. We combined the data from the two shelves with the same repellent due to the vicinity of the shelves.

The statistical tests were carried out with the open source statistical package R (R Version 2.15.1 and for the residual analyses R Version 3.0.1 for Mac).

The number of approaches per day for both gels was analyzed using a Quasi-Poisson model (function glm) with phase (three levels as described above) as the sole explanatory factor. Quasi-Poisson was used to account for overdispersion of the data. To model the time spent on the shelves per landing for each gel, we used a linear mixed model (function lmer) with the log-transformed time spent on the shelves as the outcome variable, phase as fixed factor and day as random factor. As uncertainty intervals we calculated Bayesian 95% credible intervals based on 5,000 simulations from the posterior distribution for both number of approaches and time spent on the shelves. Residual analyses included visual inspection of residual versus fitted values plots, quantile-quantile plots for both random effects and fixed effects residuals, as well as temporal autocorrelation plots. These plots indicated no serious violation of model assumptions and no substantial autocorrelation. We use the term "significant" for a fixed effect when the fitted value of one level is not included in the 95% credible interval of the other level.

Moreover, except for the approach without landing, we subdivided the possible behaviors relating to the contact of the landing pigeon with the visual gel (immediate contact, subsequent contact or no contact) into two time based categories: time spent on the experimental shelf ≤3 seconds, or >3 seconds. As pigeons have short reaction times of less than half a second, even in multi-option experiments [25], the 3 seconds that were set as the time to react to the repellents were generously determined and in favor of the effectiveness of the gels. Due to the fact that the complete repellent effect of the visual gel is supposed to have developed two or three days after gel application, we only included trial Days 4–25 in the evaluation of the affected senses. The distributor stated that the optical gel would influence the behavior of the pigeons by affecting not only the visual sense of the birds, but also the senses of smell, touch and taste. We therefore categorized the behaviors of the pigeons into seven classes to determine the affected sense in case of a positive repellent effect. We set the distant visual sense as being influenced when a pigeon approached the shelves but did not land on them. Stimulus of the near visual sense was given if the pigeon left within ≤3 seconds after it had landed on the experimental shelf and showed immediate or no contact with the gel. We defined no visual repellent effect if the pigeon landed first and had subsequent contact with the gel. For the olfactory sense we also set 3 seconds as the time between contact and flying away as the limit for a successful repellent effect, except for the subsequent contact category. Here we defined the inefficacy of the olfactory repellent effect if a pigeon landed on the shelf first and stepped into the gel afterwards. We defined a failure of the system in a tactile sense if the pigeon stood for >3 seconds in the gel. Due to the rare occurrence of events in these categories, a statistical analysis of these data was not appropriate but results were compiled in Table 1.

In terms of the animal welfare point of view we observed the consequences of the pigeons having direct contact with the gels. In addition, the effect of the gel remains transferred to other structures in the loft, and possibly also outside the loft, was described with the potential consequences for other birds.

3. Results

3.1. Contact Gel

Figure 1(a,b) shows the results of the contact gel experiment. The numbers of pigeon approaches to the shelves differed by phases. The highest number occurred to the shelves without repellent gel during the pretrial phase (70 approaches). We noted less approaches throughout trial Days 1–7 (18 approaches) and the least during trial Days 8–26 (eight approaches). During the pretrial phase, a mean of 23.3

approaches per day (14.4–37.0 Bayesian 95% credible interval), during trial Days 1–7 a mean of 3.6 (1.4–9.2) and during trial Days 8–26 a mean of 0.75 (0.18–2.95) approaches per day were recorded. The time spent on the experimental shelves during pretrial phase was significantly (or near significantly) longer than during both of the trial phases, but no significant difference occurred between trial Days 1–7 and 8–26 (Figure 1b). During the pretrial phase, the pigeons spent a mean time of 170 (77–367) seconds per landing on the shelf. Trial Days 1–7 showed a mean of 46 (16–123) seconds and trial Days 8–26 a mean of 56 (17–181) seconds per landing. Moreover, we observed only one approach during the pretrial phase that did not lead to a final landing. At this occasion the pigeon flew in the direction of an experimental shelf but turned away shortly before reaching it. In contrast, during trial phase all approaches led to a landing.

Figure 1. Feral pigeons' (**a**) mean number of approaches per day and (**b**) mean time spent on the shelf in seconds per approach for the three phases pretrial, Days 1–7 and Days 8–26 of the contact gel experiment in Basel, Switzerland, during August–October 2012. Values are means and the segments indicate Bayesian 95% credible intervals. For the mean number of approaches, with n per phase being 3, 5 and 11 recorded days, respectively, a Quasi-Poisson model was used. For the mean time spent on the shelf a mixed model with the log-transformed time on the shelf as the outcome variable (results back transformed for the graph) phase as fixed factor, and day as random factor was used with n per phase being 70, 18 and 8, respectively.

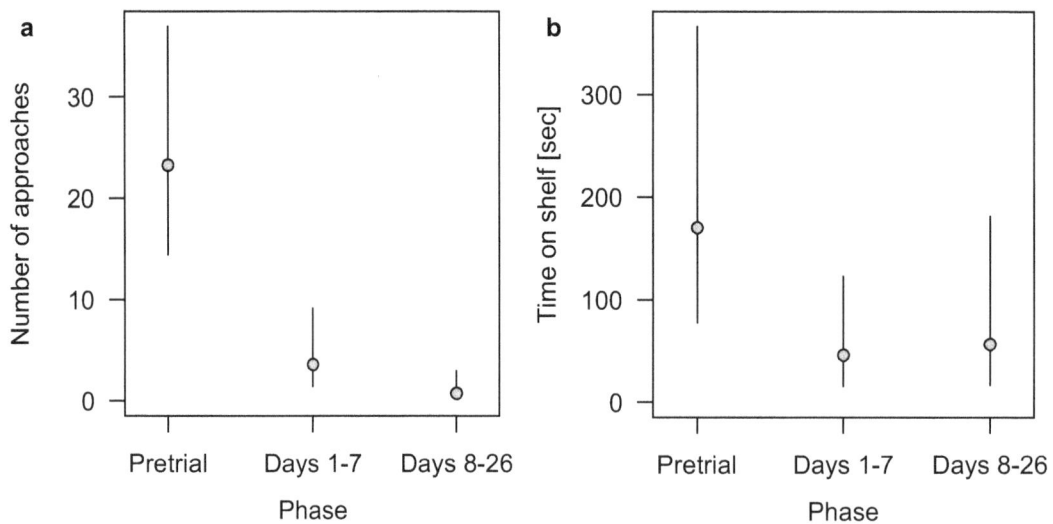

3.2. Optical Gel

During the optical gel repellent test we observed that all approaches to the experimental setup were finished with a landing. We observed a total of 56 landings during the pretrial phase. For trial Days 1–3 we monitored a total of three landings and for trial Days 4–25 a total of 13 landings. The trial phase showed a significant decrease in landings per day compared to the pretrial phase (Figure 2a). During the pretrial phase we detected a mean of 18.6 (12.0–28.9) landings per day, during trial Days 1–3 a mean of 1.53 (0.23–10.45), and during trial Days 4–25 a mean of 1.01 (0.40–2.44). We recorded no difference between trial Days 1–3 and 4–25.

Figure 2b shows that during the pretrial phase, when the shelves were not prepared with the optical gel, the pigeons spent significantly more time on the shelves per pigeon landing than during the trial phases. We observed a mean time spent on the shelves per landing of 158 (66–383) seconds during the pretrial phase, a mean of 11 (0.4–112) seconds for trial Days 1–3 and a mean of 14 (4.5–37) seconds for trial Days 4–25. There was no significant difference between the two trial phases.

Figure 2. Feral pigeons' (**a**) mean number of landings per day and (**b**) mean time spent on the shelf in seconds per landing for the three phases pretrial, Days 1–3 and Days 4–25 of the optical gel experiment in Basel, Switzerland, during August–October 2012. Values are means and the segments indicate Bayesian 95% credible intervals. For the mean number of landings, with n per phase being 3, 2 and 13 recorded days, respectively, a Quasi-Poisson model was used. For the mean time spent on the shelf, a mixed model with the log-transformed time on the shelf as the outcome variable (results back transformed for the graph), phase as fixed factor, and day as random factor was used with n per phase being 56, 3 and 13, respectively.

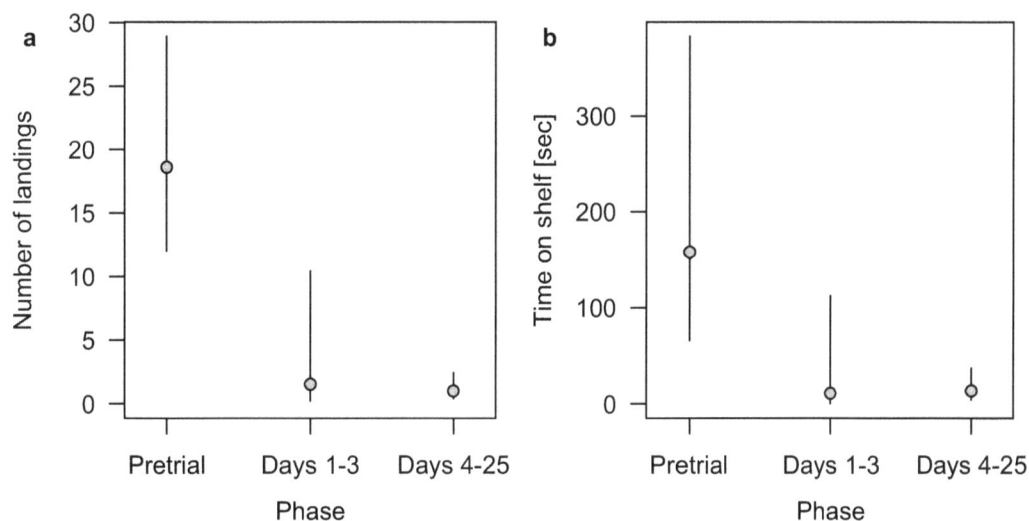

We summarized the behaviors of the pigeons to the optical gel during trial days 4–25 into seven categories to analyze which sense could have been influenced by the aversive signal (Table 1). All observed 13 approaches led to a landing and all of the stays on the protected shelves lasted >3 seconds.

Table 1. Number of behavioral responses of feral pigeons to the tested optical gel on trial Days 4–25 with determination of the senses appealed to in Basel, Switzerland, during August–October 2012. *f*, far; *p*, possible.

Behavioral response	*n*	Appealed senses
Approach without landing	0	Visual (*f*)
Landing, immediate contact, ≤3 sec	0	Visual, tactile, olfactory
Landing, immediate contact, >3 sec	7	No visual, no tactile, no olfactory
Landing, subsequent contact, ≤3sec	0	No visual, tactile (*p*), no olfactory
Landing, subsequent contact, >3 sec	4	No visual, no tactile, no olfactory,
Landing, no contact, ≤3 sec	0	Visual, olfactory
Landing, no contact, >3 sec	2	No visual, no olfactory

When testing the emission of the optical gel, a maximum at 357 nm was found. This demonstrates that the product did emit in the ultraviolet light range, which covers wavelengths of 100 nm until 380 nm.

As to the animal welfare point of view we could observe several pigeons stepping into the gels, either directly when landing onto the experimental shelves or subsequently after landing next to the shelves. Already after a short period of time, both gels looked rather unesthetic and messy due to a variety of insects, feathers and dirt that become stuck in the repellents either directly or in the remains on the shelves (Figure 3).

Figure 3. Appearance of the tactile gel (**a**) and the optical gel (**b**) after 23 days of application. Due to the adhesive effect numerous insects, feathers, dust and feces became stuck in the gels. The gluey optical gel got stuck on the wall underneath the experimental shelf when the pigeons stepped into the repellent and flew off pulling long adhesive strings. These remains were extremely difficult to remove.

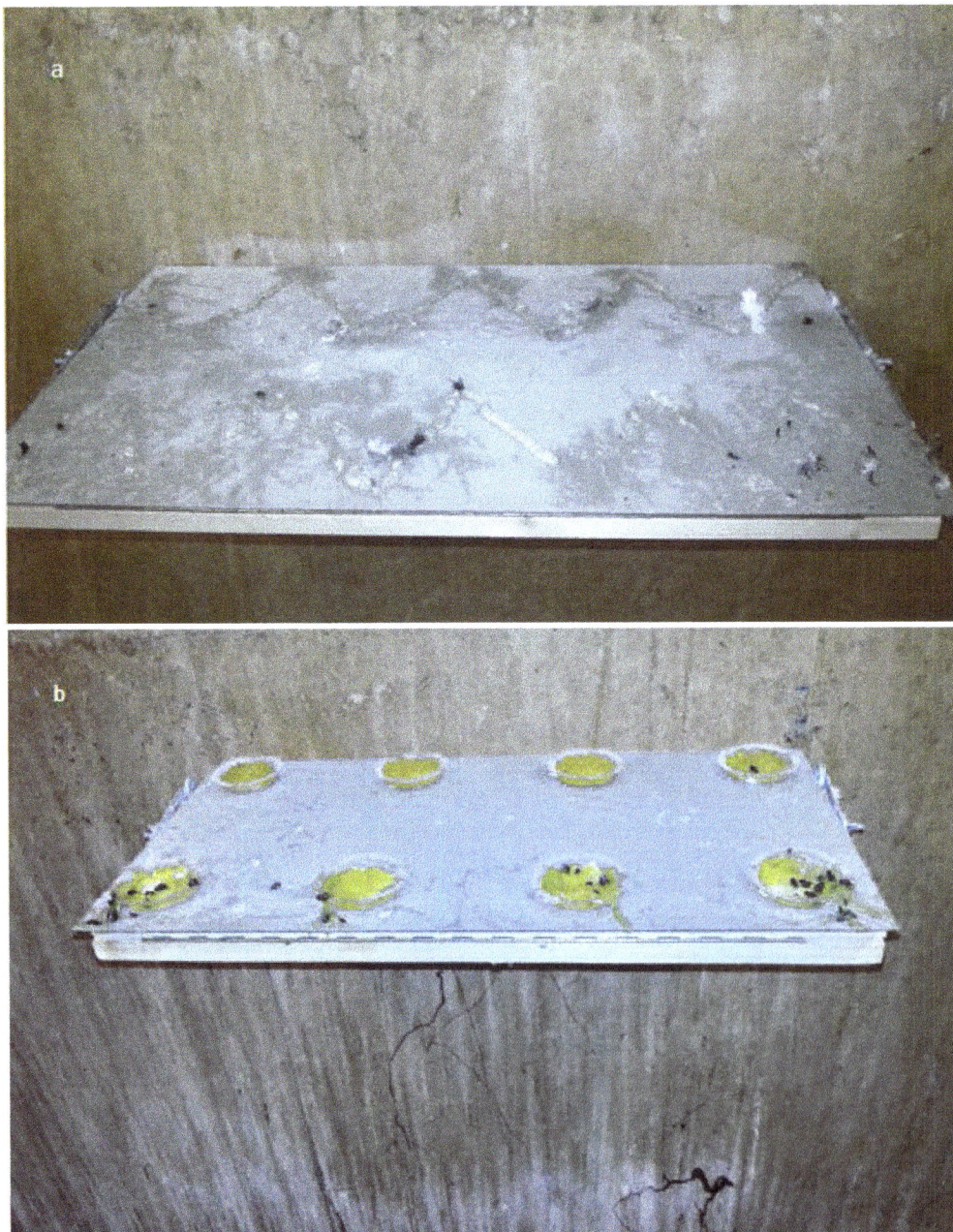

While the tactile gel is rather harmless to pigeons regarding its stickiness, the optical gel is of extremely adhesive texture. Here, the possibility of gluing of plumage is definitely given. In addition, it was observed that birds transferred the gels, especially the optical one, to numerous other structures into the loft. Due to the extremely gluey structure of the optical gel, the birds pulled long strings when they stepped into the gel and flew off (Figure 3b). These strings got stuck not only to the experimental shelves, but also to the walls, the ground and were transferred to divers other areas in the loft, as for example the nesting boxes. We can not ensure that the gel was being transferred to other areas outside the loft, but this option seems likely when looking at the numerous traces of gel being spread all over the loft. When cleaning the loft, it was extremely difficult to entirely remove the gel remains. Even strong cleaning agents were used, but some adhesive residues could not be completely removed.

4. Discussion

Both gels showed a restricted repellent effect by reducing the number of approaches of feral pigeons and their time spent on the experimental shelves per landing, but the claimed complete effectiveness, meaning a reduction of the number of birds using the protected structures by 100%, was not observed.

4.1. Contact Gel

The number of approaches during the contact gel experiment decreased constantly over the trial phases. The time spent on the shelves decreased initially, but increased again slightly during trial Days 8–26. We suspect this could be due to initiating habituation. The chance of new birds entering the loft was very low. Techniques such as tactile repellents are recognized to be of limited use because the learned avoidance of the unpleasant sensation extinguishes rapidly [11]. The repellent mechanism of the product tested is supposedly based on a slight irritation of the birds by means of capsaicin, the pungent element of red pepper. While capsaicin is an extremely effective irritant for mammals, birds are almost totally insensitive to it [13,15,16,26,27]. For this reason, a claimed sensory reaction to the gel, as stated by the distributor, is not expected. Instead, we attribute the observed repellent effect as a result of neophobia and discomfort. No complete avoidance of the experimental shelves was observed after a week of gel application. The pigeons rather appeared to get used to the new substance. They often flew onto the treated surface and stood in the repellent, which led to a constant removal of the gel (Figure 3a). Due to this contact with the gel, feces, dirt and feathers were regularly transferred onto the experimental shelves, masking any tactile effect. In addition, numerous insects also became stuck in the gel. Even though the sticky effect of the tactile repellent did not appear to be dangerous for the pigeons, any adhesive effect would make the gluing of plumage possible [12] and therefore contradicts animal welfare. When the birds preen themselves, they possibly disperse the gel even further over and into their plumage. The gel can also be transferred onto other structures and potentially affect non-target, perchance even protected, species.

A repellent effect was detected, but a complete effectiveness of the gel, which is necessary in feral pigeon proofing, is missing. Additionally, the gel has an unpleasant esthetic aspect and a limited life span due to fouling with dust, insects, feathers and feces. Furthermore, the possibility of gluing of plumage and of affecting other structures and non-target birds is given. Due to these reasons, we cannot recommend the tested tactile gel repellent.

4.2. Optical Gel

The optical gel repellent led to a decrease in landings over the trial phases. The time spent on the experimental shelves per landing was initially reduced but then increased again slightly during trial Days 4–25. The gel failed to achieve complete effectiveness since the pigeons still flew onto the treated surfaces after more than 3 days of gel application. According to the distributor, the product tested is able to repel birds visually because it is perceived as fire in their ultraviolet visual spectrum. In addition, the distributor claimed a reinforced repellent effect caused by natural oils that should be abhorrent on an olfactory, gustatory and tactile basis. Even though the effectiveness of certain repellents can be improved by additional sensory cues [28], this gel did not achieve complete avoidance of the perch area after three days of application and thus failed to prove the essential full effectiveness. According to the distributer's statement, the gel is seen as fire by the birds. Despite the fact that pigeons are certainly sensitive to ultraviolet light [29] and therefore could possibly perceive the gel as fire, one wonders how a pigeon should be familiar with fire and associate it with danger given the lack of experience. An inborn avoidance of ultraviolet light and fire lacks any evidence. The emission measurement of the optical gel showed that the gel did emit in the ultraviolet light range. However, only flames at temperatures hotter than 2,500 °C contain ultraviolet parts of the light spectrum. A normal fire by contrast does not contain ultraviolet light [30]. The reasoning of the birds seeing the optical gel as fire could therefore not be reconstructed. In addition, the effect of an outdoor use of the gel in the dark, as well as an indoor use without a supplementary artificial light source, remains questionable. According to our tests, it is not possible that the optical gel owns a repellent effect due to ultraviolet light emission. We suggest instead that the observed change in landings and time spent on the experimental shelves is due to other factors.

Furthermore, we observed a unique event during which a pigeon landed directly into one of the dishes and pecked into the gel repellent after about two seconds. This was repeated twice 13 seconds later. This observation suggests that the gel has no negative effect on the gustatory sense of a pigeon. In addition, all of the 13 approaches led to a landing and the pigeons stood longer than three seconds on the protected shelves or even directly in the gel. This further suggests that the gel does not work on the above-mentioned senses of pigeons.

5. Conclusions

Overall, we conclude that both gels showed a repellent effect, but failed to display the complete effectiveness that is unquestionably essential for a successful feral pigeon management. Our results indicate that capsaicin is ineffective in feral pigeon repellent systems. This is consistent with several other studies and the fact that pigeons are not irritated by capsaicin due to their lack of capsaicin-receptors [13,15,16,26,27]. The primarily observed repulsive effect of both gels is presumably due to neophobia, discomfort and the reduction of space on the shelves. For our second trial phase, we observed a slight, yet statistically not significant, increase in the time spent on the shelves per landing for both gels. Such a fading effect of the repellent is most likely to occur if this effect is based on startle responses due to neophobia. If the relevant stimuli are presented more than a few times, the animals desired to be repelled get accustomed to them [13,31].

As previously shown [19], young and inexperienced birds in particular landed repeatedly on the protected structures. Thus a test run was cancelled prematurely because the chance of nestlings getting directly into contact with the gels was too high. Especially the optical gel had an extreme adhesive effect, which could possibly lead to severe gluing of plumage of any bird as it already occurred with other so-called safe bird repellents [32]. Even weeks after the end of the study, we detected sticky remains of the repellents in the loft. This would definitely leave negative esthetic residues on surfaces if applied onto building facades, possibly causing even more damage than the pigeon droppings themselves. Given the possibility of young birds and also non-target birds coming into contact with the adhesive gels and the fact that any stickiness, even if relatively harmless, contradicts animal welfare, we can not approve the gels.

In our experimental situation, the treated shelves were not particularly attractive to the birds because the pigeon loft offered enough room where the repellents could be avoided. The fact that the pigeons still landed on the treated surfaces shows that even pigeons with low motivation can easily surmount the tested repellents. Summarizing, both gels seem to have only an ineffective, non-permanent repellent effect. Nevertheless, only repellents reducing the number of birds using the treated structures by 100% are effective systems. Therefore the tested products are not recommendable for a successful feral pigeon management.

Systems based on exclusion and mechanical barriers still remain the most reliable repellents. However, the best way of efficiently coping with the pigeon problem in our cities seems to be the reduction of the pigeon population, and this can only be achieved by reducing the food supply of the birds [2].

Acknowledgments

We thank Andreas Ochsenbein for technical assistance and support. Pius Korner-Nievergelt helped with the statistical analysis and Henner Sandman provided information about ultraviolet light. Jonas Schönle performed the emission measurements. Trevor Petney kindly checked the English.

Conflicts of Interest

The authors declare no conflict of interest.

References

1. Haag-Wackernagel, D. *Die Taube*; Verlag Schwabe & Co. AG: Basel, Switzerland, 1998.
2. Haag, D. Ein Beitrag zur Ökologie der Stadttaube. Ph.D. Thesis, University of Basel, Basel, Switzerland, 1984.
3. Haag-Wackernagel, D. Gesundheitsgefährdungen durch die Straßentaube *Columba livia*: Krankheiten. *Amtstierärztlicher Dienst und Lebensmittelkontrolle* **2006**, *4*, 262–272.
4. Haag-Wackernagel, D. Gesundheitsgefährdungen durch die Straßentaube *Columba livia*: Parasiten. *Amtstierärztlicher Dienst und Lebensmittelkontrolle* **2008**, *3*, 174–188.
5. Haag-Wackernagel, D.; Moch, H. Health hazards posed by feral pigeons. *J. Infect.* **2004**, *48*, 307–313.

6.   Feare, C.J. Humane control of urban birds. In *Humane Control of Land Mammals and Birds: Proceedings of a Symposium at the University of Surrey, Guildford, Surrey, England, 17th to 19th September, 1984*; Britt, D.P., Ed.; Universities Federation for Animal Welfare: Hertfordshire, UK, 1985; pp. 50–62.

7.   Vogel, C.; Vogel, M.; Detering, W.; Löffler, M. *Tauben*; Deutscher Landwirtschaftsverlag: Berlin, Germany, 1992; p. 355.

8.   Haag-Wackernagel, D. Strassentauben am Gebäude. In *Handbuch Gebäude-Schadstoffe und Gesunde Innenraumluft*; Zwiener, G., Lange, F.-M., Eds.; Erich Schmidt Verlag: Berlin, Germany, 2012; pp. 597–633.

9.   Zucconi, S.; Galavotti, S.; Deserti, R. I colombi in ambiente urbano—Sintesi del progetto di ricerca Nomisma. *Disinfestazione* **2003**, *November/December*, 9–22.

10. Pimentel, D.; Zuniga, R.; Morrison, D. Update on the environmental and economic costs associated with alien-invasive species in the United States. *Ecol. Econ.* **2005**, *52*, 273–288.

11. Clark, L. Review of bird repellents. In Proceedings of the Eighteenth Vertebrate Pest Conference, University of California Davis, Davis, CA, USA, 1998; pp. 330–337.

12. Wormuth, H.-J.; Lagoni, N. Taubenabwehr und Tierschutz—Verwendung sogenannter Repellents. *Der praktische Tierarzt* **1985**, *3*, 242–244.

13. Mason, J.R. Overview of controls: Why they work and how they function: Repellents. In *Wildlife Damage Management for Natural Resource Managers*; Nolte, D.L., Wagner, K.K., Eds.; Western Forestry and Conservation Association: Portland, OR, USA, 1997; pp. 11–16.

14. Mason, J.R.; Clark, L. Avian repellents: Options, modes of action, and economic considerations. In *Repellents in Wildlife Management*; Mason, J.R., Ed.; Colorado State University Press: Fort Collins, CO, USA, 1997; pp. 371–391.

15. Clark, L. Physiological, ecological, and evolutionary bases for the avoidance of chemical irritants by birds. In *Current Ornithology*; Nolan, V., Ketterson, E.D., Eds.; Plenum Press: New York, NY, USA, 1998; Volume 14, pp. 1–37.

16. Mason, J.R. Mammal repellents: Options and considerations for development. In Proceedings of the Eighteenth Vertebrate Pest Conference, University of California Davis, Davis, CA, USA, 1998; pp. 325–329.

17. Stevens, G.R.; Clark, L. Bird repellents: Development of avian-specific tear gases for resolution of human-wildlife conflicts. *Int. Biodeterior. Biodegrad.* **1998**, *42*, 153–160.

18. Giunchi, D.; Albores-Barajas, Y.V.; Baldaccini, N.E.; Vanni, L.; Soldatini, C. Feral Pigeons: Problems, Dynamics and Control Methods. In *Integrated Pest Management and Pest Control— Current and Future Tactics*; Larramendy, M.L., Soloneski, S., Eds.; InTech Open Science: Rijeka, Croatia, 2012; pp. 215–240.

19. Haag-Wackernagel, D. Behavioural responses of the feral pigeon (Columbidae) to deterring systems. *Folia Zool.* **2000**, *49*, 101–114.

20. Avery, M.L. Avian repellants. In *Encyclopedia of Agrochemicals*; Plimmer, J.R., Gammon, D.W., Ragsdale, N.N., Eds.; John Wiley & Sons: Hoboken, NJ, USA, 2003; Volume 1, pp. 122–128.

21. Haag-Wackernagel, D.; Geigenfeind, I. Protecting buildings against feral pigeons. *Eur. J. Wildl. Res.* **2008**, *54*, 715–721.

22. Alderson, C.; Greene, A. Bird-Deterrence Technology for Historic Buildings. *Assoc. Preserv. Technol. (APT) Bull.* **1995**, *26*, 18–30.

23. Rose, E.; Nagel, P.; Haag-Wackernagel, D. Spatio-temporal use of the urban habitat by feral pigeons (*Columba livia*). *Behav. Ecol. Sociobiol.* **2006**, *60*, 242–254.

24. Jancsó, N.; Jancsó-Gábor, A.; Szolcsányi, J. Direct evidence for neurogenic inflammation and its prevention by denervation and by pretreatment with capsaicin. *Br. J. of Pharmacol. Chemother.* **1967**, *31*, 138–151.

25. Vickrey, C.; Neuringer, A. Pigeon reaction time, Hick's law, and intelligence. *Psychon. Bull. Rev.* **2000**, *7*, 284–291.

26. Szolcsányi, J.; Sann, H.; Pierau, F.-K. Nociception in pigeons is not impaired by capsaicin. *Pain* **1986**, *27*, 247–260.

27. Mason, J.R.; Bean, N.J.; Shah, P.S.; Clark, L. Taxon-specific differences in responsiveness to capsaicin and several analogues: correlates between chemical structure and behavioral aversiveness. *J. Chem. Ecol.* **1991**, *17*, 2539–2551.

28. Mason, J.R. Avoidance of methiocarb-poisoned apples by Red-winged Blackbirds. *J. Wildl. Manag.* **1989**, *53*, 836–840.

29. Kreithen, M.L.; Eisner, T. Ultraviolet light detection by the homing pigeon. *Nature* **1978**, *272*, 347–348.

30. Sandmann, H. University of Kiel, Kiel, Germany. Personal communication, 2013.

31. Dinetti, M. Urban Avifauna: Is it Possible to Life Together? *Vet. Res. Commun.* **2006**, *30*, 3–7.

32. Jensen, E. Sticky situation—"Safe" bird repellant creates horror story. Available online: http://www.urbanwildlifesociety.org/UWS/BrdCtrl/AZRpbStickyBrds.html (accessed on 19 September 2013).

Psychogenic Stress in Hospitalized Dogs: Cross Species Comparisons, Implications for Health Care, and the Challenges of Evaluation

Jessica P. Hekman [1], **Alicia Z. Karas** [2,]* and **Claire R. Sharp** [2]

[1] Department of Animal Sciences, University of Illinois at Urbana-Champaign,
    1207 West Gregory Drive, Urbana, IL 61801, USA; E-Mail: hekman2@illinois.edu

[2] Department of Clinical Sciences, Cummings School of Veterinary Medicine, Tufts University,
    200 Westboro Road, North Grafton, MA 01536, USA; E-Mail: claire.sharp@tufts.edu

* Author to whom correspondence should be addressed; E-Mail: alicia.karas@tufts.edu.

Simple Summary: The effects of stress on health outcomes in animals are well documented. Veterinary clinicians may be able to improve their patients' care by better understanding how to recognize and reduce stress in those patients. This review will describe the physiology of the mammalian stress response and known health consequences of psychogenic, rather than physical, stress; as well as methods of measuring stress in animals. While the review will address stress in a range of domestic species, it will specifically focus on dogs.

Abstract: Evidence to support the existence of health consequences of psychogenic stress has been documented across a range of domestic species. A general understanding of methods of recognition and means of mitigation of psychogenic stress in hospitalized animals is arguably an important feature of the continuing efforts of clinicians to improve the well-being and health of dogs and other veterinary patients. The intent of this review is to describe, in a variety of species: the physiology of the stress syndrome, with particular attention to the hypothalamic-pituitary-adrenal axis; causes and characteristics of psychogenic stress; mechanisms and sequelae of stress-induced immune dysfunction; and other adverse effects of stress on health outcomes. Following that, we describe general aspects of the measurement of stress and the role of physiological measures and behavioral signals that may predict stress in hospitalized animals, specifically focusing on dogs.

Keywords: stress; hospitalization; dogs

1. Introduction

In recent decades, the effects of stress on human health, and methods to reduce its prevalence, have received a great deal of attention. It is a long recognized phenomenon that husbandry and transport stress can dramatically affect animal health in livestock, and stress is beginning to be recognized as a factor in naturally occurring disease in humans [1,2]. The clinical relevance of stress in small animal veterinary patients has not been examined, but it seems likely that the impact of stress on clinical outcomes, such as survival rates or the speed of recovery from surgery, is under-appreciated. The implications that stress has for human health care outcomes and health in livestock serve as a foundation from which to extrapolate an analogous concern for our small animal veterinary patients. Reducing stress in companion animals under veterinary care is clearly important for their mental well-being, and is even more important if pharmacologic or non-pharmacologic interventions can also prevent disease or improve healthcare outcomes.

The experience of hospitalization may be expected to include several factors which are known to induce stress in veterinary species such as the dog, including separation from the primary caretaker [3], environment [4], novel stimuli [5], increased noise levels [6], and a constrained environment [7,8]. An investigation of behavior and heart rate of pre-operative hospitalized dogs suggests that these animals experience stress [9], yet there is little detail regarding the effects of such stress on health outcomes for dogs. This is likely in part due to a lack of understanding of stress by veterinary clinicians, as well as a lack of tools for accurate identification and quantification of stress in dogs. Investigation of the causes and effects of stress on the hospitalized small animal patient requires an understanding of both its physiology and pathophysiology, and of available methods of quantification in that particular species. The purpose of this review is to describe the physiology of the stress syndrome, characteristics of stressors, stress-induced immune dysfunction, and other adverse effects of stress on health using a cross-species approach. Following that, general aspects of the measurement of stress and the role of behavioral signals that may predict it are described, specifically focusing on dogs.

2. Physiology of the Stress Syndrome

The stress response is a normal part of daily life, and is only harmful when triggered too intensely or for too long [10,11]. Peripheral expression of the stress response is modulated via two systems, the sympatho-adreno-medullary (SAM) axis and the hypothalamic-pituitary-adrenal (HPA) axis.

The SAM axis mediates the well-known "fight or flight" response, an initial, rapid response to an immediate stressor. Activation of the sympathetic nervous system and subsequent release of catecholamines (epinephrine and norephinephrine) from sympathetic nerve terminals and the adrenal medulla results in a state of physiologic readiness for response. Manifestations of SAM axis activation include mydriasis, increased heart rate, increased blood pressure, cutaneous vasoconstriction, an alert state, and increased plasma glucose and free fatty acid concentrations [12].

A slower response to a stressor, with effects in minutes to hours or days, is mediated by activation of the HPA axis leading to the release of glucocorticoids (GCs) from the adrenal cortex. This endocrine portion of the mammalian stress response originates in the hypothalamus, with release of corticotropin releasing hormone and arginine vasopressin. These hormones in turn stimulate the release of adrenocorticotropic hormone from the pituitary gland, resulting in the production and release of GCs from the adrenal glands. Peripherally circulating GCs, cortisol and corticosterone, provide negative feedback to this system [12]. Glucocorticoids influence a large number of metabolic processes, including protein, glucose, and fatty acid metabolism, and immune function [13], and can induce a catabolic state [14], while corticotropin releasing hormone suppreses gastro-intestinal motility [15,16] and arginine vasopressin regulates the glomerular filtration rate (GFR), cAMP generation, and fluid balance [17]. Acting jointly, these hormones can also influence growth, thyroid function, and reproduction [18].

3. Classification and Causes of Stress

Stress can be classified in a variety of ways, and different classifications of stress may have different consequences for health outcomes. Stress can be acute or chronic. In the laboratory setting, acute stress is sometimes defined as having a duration of less than one hour [19]. Chronic stressors in the laboratory often persist for 4–5 days, though chronic psychosocial stress in humans can last years [20]. These definitions differ from clinical perceptions of acute *versus* chronic disease, in which a disease lasting as long as several weeks may still be considered acute [21,22].

The term "stress" covers several different concepts: physiologic stress, non-physiologic or psychogenic stress, and distress [10]. Physiologic stress describes exposure to positive or negative physical, systemic, or environmental challenges that perturb the body's homeostasis. In a veterinary setting, negative physiologic stress may be induced by systemic illness, trauma, and surgery. Similarly, psychogenic stress describes exposure to psychological or social challenges which result in disruption of psychological well-being. Negative psychogenic stress in a domesticated animal may be induced by separation from a caretaker, being subjected to invasive procedures in the absence of familiar caretakers, or exposure to a novel environment [23]. Positive psychogenic stress has been less widely studied, but may be understood to refer to situations such as reunion with a caretaker or engagement in a highly anticipated game such as fetch. Negative psychogenic stressors may account for some degree of avoidable morbidity in medical care, if measures to reduce stressors exist. Both physiologic and psychogenic stress are a normal part of life, and the healthy body and mind can adapt to maintain normal function [11]. Stress becomes distress when the body cannot restore homeostasis in the face of overwhelming physiologic stress, or when overwhelming psychogenic stress threatens mental well-being [10]. When marked, stress is associated with numerous pathophysiological sequellae, ranging from poor mental to poor physical well-being. This review is concerned with negative psychogenic stress, especially as it proceeds to distress. Following the stress literature, the term "stress" will be used to refer to "distress."

Psychogenic stressors may be classified as social/non-social [24] or controllable/uncontrollable [25]. A social stressor involves aversive interactions with a hostile conspecific, such as aggressive dogs in facing cages, or separation from the attachment figure, as opposed to a nonsocial stressor, such as exposure to aversive environmental conditions, such as elevated noise levels. An uncontrollable stressor is not escapable by the animal, such as inescapable electric shock or restraint for medical procedures, as opposed to a controllable stressor, such as social stress mitigated by retreat to the rear of the cage. All of these types of stressors might be present in a veterinary medical setting; hostile conspecifics might present a social stressor, and restraint for a medical procedure might present an uncontrollable stressor. Practically, social stressors due to a lack of accommodation to canine body language and needs by their human caregiver are also uncontrollable, and are arguably widely encountered in veterinary care.

Different stressors are known to cause varying levels of activation of metabolic and endocrine responses in laboratory animals [26,27], and may also have varying consequences in hospitalized animals. For example, social stressors such as defeat in conflict with a conspecific activate the sympathetic nervous system more strongly than non-social stressors (restraint and shock) in rats [24]. Uncontrollable stressors, e.g., stressors from which the animal cannot escape and which cannot be mitigated, appear to activate the stress response more strongly across species than controllable stressors. This has been shown with escapable *versus* inescapable electric shocks in dogs [25]. Enhanced skill in assessment of and response to body language cues, as well as addressing a hospitalized animal's environmental needs, may produce an overall reduction in psychogenic stress.

4. The Effects of Stress on Health Outcomes

There is ample evidence from laboratory, clinical, and epidemiological trials demonstrating that acute and chronic psychogenic stress can result in negative consequences on both human and non-human animals, contributing to increased patient morbidity or mortality [28]. These health implications include, but are not limited to, susceptibility to infection and sepsis, impaired antibody responses to vaccination, slowed wound healing, and development of gastric ulceration [28–30]. Chronic stress from anxiety disorders is associated with shortened lifespan in dogs [31]. Outcomes of particular relevance to hospitalized animals will be discussed under the subheadings below.

4.1. Interactions between the Stress Response and the Immune System

There is a complex interplay between the stress response and the immune system, which varies based on the duration (acute or chronic), timing (before or after immune challenge), and type (social or non-social, controllable or uncontrollable) of the stressor. The balance between the immunoenhancing and immunosuppressive effects of stress is complex, and any stressor may theoretically be immunoenhancing or immunosuppressive in a particular individual, based on the aforementioned variables.

The initial stress response to a psychogenic stressor or an injury is often immunoenhancing and pro-inflammatory [32]. Acute stress enhances T lymphocyte responsiveness and appropriate differentiation into T helper 1 (Th1) or T helper 2 (Th2) lymphocytes [19,33]. Increased endogenous GC production associated with acute stress may result in a "stress leukogram," characterized by a peripheral neutrophilia, lymphopenia, eosinopenia, and monocytosis due to redistribution and increased trafficking of white blood cells [34]. Circulating natural killer cell numbers may also increase, and the levels of both pro- and anti-inflammatory cytokines are altered [35,36]. Taken together, these changes prepare the immune system for an impending challenge, such as microbial invasion.

As time passes and an acute stressor becomes chronic, the effects of the stress response on the immune system may shift from immunoenhancement to immunosuppression. Glucocorticoids can inappropriately suppress the Th1 response and enhance the Th2 response [33]. Chronic stress can also be associated with leukopenia, lymphopenia, and reduced leukocyte phagocytic capacity [37]. These immunosuppressive and anti-inflammatory properties of the chronic stress response may be adaptive to limit systemic inflammation while permitting a controlled, localized inflammatory response to injury or infection, or to shift from the innate immune response to the adaptive immune response when the stressor is of longer duration, allowing enough time for the slower adaptive response to be effective [32,33].

However, when activation of the stress response is exaggerated or prolonged, it may lead to inappropriate immunosuppression [38]. For example, chronic stress induced immunosuppression in humans can lead to increased susceptibility to infection and neoplasia and decreased response to vaccination [28,39]. In mice, chronic restraint and acoustic stress results in decreased ability to eliminate bacterial infection associated with mild peritonitis [38].

The timing of the stressor is also important. The immunoenhancing effects of acute stress are best realized when the stressor is timed to occur just before immune challenge. When a stressor occurs after the onset of an immune response, the stressor is more likely to be suppressive, even in the acute setting [19].

In addition to the duration and timing of the stressor, the type of stressor may also affect the pro-*versus* anti-inflammatory consequences of that stress. For example, social disruption stress in mice is pro-inflammatory, and presumed to be an adaptive response, since it is often associated with physical conflict resulting in wounds [40].

Hospitalized animals may be exposed to both acute and chronic stressors of a variety of types, including social, nonsocial, uncontrollable, and controllable. The interactions of immunoenhancing acute stressors *versus* immunosuppressing chronic stressors may be difficult to predict. However, as stressors associated with hospitalization of companion animals often occur after the challenge that initially prompted presentation of the animal to the veterinary hospital, they may be expected to be immunosuppressive, not immunoenhancing. Similarly, as the animal's time in the hospital extends, the stress of hospitalization becomes more likely to act as chronic rather than acute stress, and therefore becomes more likely to suppress rather than enhance the immune response.

4.2. Response to Vaccination

Acute stress, on the order of minutes or hours, is immunoenhancing, so that stress may essentially serve as a natural adjuvant when it occurs at the time of vaccination [19] and has been shown in mice to induce a long-lasting increase in immunity [41] through enhancement of both the adaptive and innate arms of the immune system [42]. Timing is essential, however, because psychogenic stressors occurring after vaccination have been associated with a poorer antibody response [43], and a stressor which becomes chronic may suppress rather than enhance immune activity [19]. These beneficial effects appear to be mediated by endogenous glucocorticoids in physiologic, not pharmacologic, concentrations [19].

4.3. Susceptibility to Sepsis

Stress may influence an animal's susceptibility to sepsis. In sepsis, an exaggerated systemic response to infection occurs, which results in increased mortality and may be more damaging than the original infection [40]. Studies in mice suggest that increased GC concentrations due to psychogenic stress might provide protection against sepsis due to the immunosuppressive effects of GCs, or might increase susceptibility to sepsis due to increased GC resistance, depending on the effects of different stressor types [13,44]. It is not known whether stress might increase or decrease susceptibility to sepsis in hospitalized veterinary patients.

4.4. Wound Healing

In humans, both acute and chronic psychogenic stress can negatively affect wound healing, even when activated for as short a time as several hours or days, as may be the case in hospitalized animals [45]. Chronic psychogenic stressors shown to affect wound healing in humans include examination stress, care taking for dementia patients, and marital stress [46]. Additionally, greater amounts of stress perceived pre-operatively in humans predict slower wound healing [45]. Therefore, psychogenic stress during hospitalization might be expected to affect wound healing in veterinary patients with traumatic wounds and surgical incisions.

4.5. Gastrointestinal System

Stress has been shown in humans and in laboratory animals to induce the development of stomach ulcers, particularly in conjunction with pathogens such as Helicobacter pylori, or non-steroidal anti-inflammatory drugs [47]. Chronic stress is also associated with the exacerbation of inflammatory bowel disease in humans [48], and stressful environment and anxious personality traits are associated with chronic idiopathic large-bowel disease in dogs [49]. Dogs undergoing significant physiological stress in the form of the physical exertion of a sled race are at increased risk of developing gastric lesions [50]. In addition to physiological stress, sled dogs are arguably exposed to psychogenic stress in the form of exposure to unfamiliar environments, interactions with unfamiliar conspecifics, and the race itself. Similarly, hospitalized animals are exposed to physiologic stressors, in the form of illness or trauma, in addition to psychogenic stressors. However, effects of hospitalization stress on gastrointestinal function in dogs have not yet been investigated.

4.6. Cardiovascular System

The detrimental effects of psychogenic stress on cardiovascular function in humans and laboratory animals are well recognized. Acute social stress increases T-wave alternans in normal dogs, and has triggered atrial fibrillation in humans [51,52]. Acute psychogenic stress is associated with hypercoagulability and thrombotic tendencies in humans, which is exacerbated in subjects who are also undergoing chronic stress [53,54]. Additionally, chronic psychogenic stress is associated with coronary artery disease and hypertension in humans, and increased risk of cardiovascular disease occurrence, morbidity, and mortality [55–57]. It is not known at this time how stress affects the cardiovascular systems of hospitalized animals with or without heart disease.

5. Quantification of Stress

Although the effects of stress on health outcomes have been well studied in humans and animal models, little work has been done to evaluate the effects of different stressors on health outcomes in hospitalized animals with naturally occurring disease. It is likely that, as in other species, effects of stress on specific health outcomes in veterinary patients will vary depending on the duration, timing, and type of stressor(s). In order to better understand how stress affects hospitalized veterinary patients, reliable measurement tools are essential. As various markers of stress can be species specific, the following section focuses primarily on the dog.

Quantification of stress is difficult. Both physiological and behavioral measures have been used to quantify psychogenic stress. However, both approaches have drawbacks, and results may be challenging to interpret. Theoretically, psychogenic stress may be objectively evaluated by measuring the circulating concentrations of SAM or HPA axis hormones, or associated physiologic parameters, such as heart rate variability as a representation of autonomic tone. In practice, no single hormone or physiological response is ideal for measuring psychogenic stress, and it has been suggested that multiple parameters should be used simultaneously to improve accuracy [10]. There are no known physiological measurements of stress which can serve as specific markers of distress; measuring stress is made difficult by confounding factors, such as measurements that describe the function of the immune system in addition to characterizing the stress response. Behavioral measures of stress suffer from similar non-specificity, and are in many ways less well understood than physiological measures.

5.1. Physiological Measures of Stress

Physiological measurements of stress include assessment of the HPA axis (usually cortisol measurement), salivary immunoglobulin (Ig)A (sIgA), and the neutrophil:lymphocyte (N:L) ratio. The benefits and limitations of each of these are discussed below. Additionally, Table 1 summarizes some physiological measures of stress in regards to their invasiveness, the time period that they reflect, and daily variation.

Table 1. Physiological measurements of stress in dogs.

Type	Invasiveness	Time period reflected	Daily variation
Plasma cortisol	Moderate	3–40 minutes	High
Salivary cortisol	Low	4–40 minutes	High
Urinary cortisol	None	6–12 hours	Low
Salivary IgA	Low	0–30 minutes	High
N:L ratio	Moderate	Hours	Low
HRV	Moderate	Hours	High

5.1.1. The HPA Axis

Measurement of HPA axis activity through concentrations of GCs such as cortisol and corticosterone is the most widely used hormonal measurement of psychogenic stress, and is commonly used in humans and dogs [58–60]. Cortisol concentrations in the plasma, saliva, or urine have been shown to significantly increase in dogs 15–30 minutes after the onset of a stressor, indicating increased HPA axis activation [61]. Because blood collection is moderately invasive, many animals will display increased cortisol concentrations after immobilization and venipuncture. However, cortisol secretion in response to collection does not affect the values in dogs if venipuncture and collection can be completed in less than 3 minutes, or if saliva collection can be completed in less than 4 minutes [62]. Salivary cortisol concentrations are frequently used in stress studies of dogs because they are strongly correlated with plasma cortisol, are less invasive, and require less training of the handler performing the collection [59,63]. Urine contains both cortisol and its metabolites, and may be collected non-invasively. Urine cortisol:creatinine ratios provide a summary of HPA axis activity over several hours, and are therefore more useful for measurement of chronic stress than of HPA axis response to an acute stressor [64].

The evaluation of HPA axis activation by means of cortisol concentration measurement has multiple limitations. Measurement of cortisol activity reflects physical and/or psychological arousal, and therefore is not a specific measurement of psychogenic stress. The level of psychogenic distress experienced by an individual may be only moderately associated with cortisol concentrations, due to the intricate relationship of HPA axis function and metabolic demands [59,65]. In fact, activation of the HPA axis may indicate positive stress rather than distress, as it is activated in dogs after time in the dog park [66] or in sled dogs anticipating a race [67]. Moreover, due to the degree of variability in cortisol concentrations between individuals, no reliable species reference ranges exist, and basal concentrations must be evaluated with reference to a control group [68]. Daily variability in cortisol concentrations is such that sampling the same animal on multiple days is recommended where possible [62]. Additionally, samples should be obtained at the same time of day to avoid possible diurnal variability [69]. These samples may be affected by daily experience, including sleep patterns, meal content, and recent exercise [69–71].

To some extent, study design can mitigate the issue of variability in cortisol concentrations, by pairing similar subjects in statistical analysis, taking multiple samples, taking samples at the same time of day, and by limiting the variety of ages, breeds, and life experience where possible. However, cortisol alone is not a highly reliable measurement of stress. Despite its common use, it has proven to be a problematic tool at best, due to its extreme inter- and intra-individual variability.

5.1.2. Salivary Immunoglobulin (Ig) A

Salivary immunoglobulin(Ig)A (sIgA) is a well-known marker of stress in humans [72]. sIgA concentrations have been shown to negatively correlate with cortisol concentrations in dogs, and have been used to evaluate both acute and chronic stress in dogs [73,74]. Limitations of using sIgA concentrations to assess stress are that they change rapidly, will decline immediately after the presentation of a stressor, have significant diurnal variation, and may fail to distinguish between physiologic and psychogenic stress [73,75]. Because sIgA concentrations significantly correlate with plasma cortisol concentrations, they may be subject to similar variation, though causes of variability of sIgA are not as well described in domesticated animals as are causes of cortisol variability [74].

5.1.3. Neutrophil: Lymphocyte (N:L) Ratio

Because both acute and chronic stress are known to be associated with neutrophilia and lymphopenia, an increased neutrophil:lymphocyte (N:L) ratio has been used as a marker of stress in human and veterinary studies, including studies in dogs [8,76]. Using the N:L ratio has the advantage of a several-hour time delay from the onset of the stressor, so that it may be used to measure baseline stress levels in dogs who have recently arrived at a veterinary hospital.

Limitations of the N:L are similar to those of GC concentrations, in that it cannot distinguish between physiologic and psychogenic stress and is invasive; therefore, this marker may not be appropriate for all studies [76]. This ratio suffers from less variability than cortisol concentrations, but is correspondingly less responsive in the short term to the effects of very acute stressors [76]. Additionally, its use in veterinary studies of stress is much less common and less well understood than the use of cortisol.

5.1.4. Heart Rate and Heart Rate Variability

Sympathetic nervous system activation during psychogenic stress results in increased heart rate, which has been used to assess acute stress in dogs [3,77–79]. However, heart rate elevation has been found to be a non-specific marker of distress, increasing in cases of positive and negative stress, as well as with increased motor activity [3,77,79]. Heart rate ordinarily varies over time due to the prevailing balance of parasympathetic and sympathetic nervous system input. During stressful events, heart rate variability (HRV) declines as the heart rate remains mostly elevated, and this parameter can be measured and interpreted. Decreased HRV has been shown to be present in dogs which may be suffering from stress due to hospitalization [9]. Heart rate variability has also been used as a marker of acute stress in humans [80] and lab animals [24], and may prove valuable as a marker of acute stress in dogs. Heart rate variability measurement requires continuous monitoring, typically accomplished via attachment of telemetry equipment [78,79], but more simple and feasible methods developed for human athletes hold promise for studies of stress in dogs [81,82]. Ideally, dogs should be acclimated to wearing telemetry devices, in order to avoid the confounding of the response to the experimental stressor with a reaction to the equipment [77].

5.1.5. Additional Physiologic Measures

ACTH, norepinephrine, and epinephrine [8,83] have been used as biomarkers of stress in dogs, but only rarely. Additional measures of physiologic change have been documented in dogs post-surgically, including decreased prolactin, monocytosis, eosinopenia, and increased C-reactive protein and haptoglobin [23], but these measures have not been used as biomarkers of stress in dogs.

5.1.6. Limitations of Physiologic Measurements of Stress

An understanding of the limitations of measurement of physiologic changes to evaluate psychogenic stress is important when designing stress studies using these measurements. What one individual experiences as a stressor, another may not, and stimuli which evoke a stress response in one individual may not do so in another. A standardized stress stimulation tool in humans, the Trier Social Stress

Test, produces a stress response measurable with cortisol in only 70–80% of tested individuals [84]. Similarly, a hospital environment triggering a stress response in one dog may not do so in another individual coming from a comparatively more stimulating or stressful home environment. In other words, though physiologic changes are likely to reflect an animal's distress, prediction of what constitutes a stressor for a specific individual may be difficult if the animal's prior history is unknown. Conclusions from studies using purpose-bred dogs of uniform age, breed, gender, and life experience should be applied to pet dogs, a population which might vary in all of those parameters, only with caution. On the other hand, studies on pet dogs may be confounded by variability in such a large number of parameters that the necessary sample size to reach statistical significance may be much larger than for uniform populations.

5.2. Behavioral Markers of Stress in Dogs

Behavioral measures of stress have been used to inform interpretation of physiological markers of stress such as cortisol concentrations or heart rate, and are non-invasive [4,58,60,64]. However, behavior may be difficult to interpret, and may not be constant for different stressors [85]. In one study of stress in dogs moved to a new kennel environment, behaviors thought to be associated with stress showed no correlation with urinary cortisol concentrations [60]. The interpretation of individual behaviors may be contextual, so that behaviors may be linked to stress in some situations but not others. Oral activity such as lip licking increases after some acute stressors, including pulling the dog's head down by a rope, opening an umbrella, or pressing the dog down to the floor [86]. However, oral activity does not increase after other acute stressors, such as a loud sound or the presentation of a moving toy car [60]. Similarly, paw lifting is increased in dogs subjected to austere housing compared to dogs with more enriched housing, but not in dogs introduced to an animal shelter [60,85]. Therefore, stress behaviors cannot be grouped into categories such as "behaviors in response to acute stress" or "behaviors in response to housing stress," but must be considered for a particular environment.

5.3. The Need for Behavioral Stress Assessment Instruments for Hospitalized Dogs

Hospitalization represents a predictable set of stressors, including separation from the caretaker and exposure to novel surroundings, which may have an impact on the outcome of medical treatment. If behaviors were determined to correlate positively or negatively with cortisol concentrations or other physiologic markers, generation of stress assessment scales or instruments may be possible. Validation of scales is necessary, to guard against errors in the development process, and to ensure reproducibility.

Validated behavioral instruments have been used to assess and study other states in dogs, such as acute pain, postoperative pain, and pain from osteoarthritis [86–88]. Pain is a state that, like stress, has no "gold standard" for detection in non-verbal beings, even experimentally, but the emergence of pain scales in veterinary medicine has enhanced the study of interventions and assessments greatly in recent years.

Published studies of stress in dogs commonly involve measurement of salivary cortisol. Due to cortisol's variability and non-specificity as a marker of stress, the addition of a second marker may increase the reliability of behavioral instruments to detect stress [10]. However, the measurement of multiple physiologic variables represents a challenge in the clinical study of patient populations, particularly when such measures may themselves perturb the state of the system being studied in the subject.

In addition to allowing the study of the effects of stress on health care outcomes, behavioral assessment may provide a useful clinical diagnostic measure. Salivary cortisol is not useful for "point of care" detection of stress levels in hospitalized patients, since measurement requires an immunoassay and strict controls. Clinical evaluation of stress levels of patients currently involves interpretation of behavior [23]. Our recent work has contributed to the literature by providing some evidence for correlation of specific behavior combinations associated with salivary cortisol in hospitalized dogs [89]; however, it was necessary to observe the dogs over a period of time (20 minutes), and this was considered too cumbersome for a useful clinical observation period. Behavior is an inexpensive and non-invasive parameter to assess, but due to its high variability and lack of understanding of the specific sources of that variability in different situations, it may be difficult to interpret [85]. Therefore, in order for behavior to be a useful indicator, there is a need for more investigation into correlations between stress markers and behavior in hospitalized dogs.

6. Conclusions

Both because of a growing recognition of its potential to affect health outcomes in humans and animals, and because the experience of psychogenic distress is unpleasant, veterinarians should recognize the importance of identification and reduction of psychogenic distress in their patients. Therefore, there is a need for investigation into methods of measurement of stress in hospitalized animals. If we can produce behavioral assessment instruments, or "stress scales," to enable identification of highly stressed patients, then this may aid in determining the extent to which negative outcomes are associated with increased stress and methods to reduce its impact on the patient. As evidence accumulates in support of the fact that psychogenic stress has important health consequences across a range of species, a general understanding on the part of clinicians, as well as investigation of its recognition and means of mitigation using validated stress assessment tools, are important features of our evolving quest to improve the well-being and health of veterinary patients.

Acknowledgments

This manuscript represents a portion of a thesis submitted by Jessica Hekman to the Tufts University Cummings School of Veterinary Medicine Department of Comparative Biomedical Sciences as partial fulfillment of the requirements for a Master of Science degree.

This project was supported by the National Center for Research Resources and the Office of Research Infrastructure Programs (ORIP) of the National Institutes of Health through Grant Number T32 RR018267.

This publication was also supported by Grant Number UL1 RR025752 from the National Center for Research Resources. Its contents are solely the responsibility of the authors and do not necessarily represent the official views of the NCRR.

Supported in part by the National Institute of Health and the U.S. Army.

Conflicts of Interest

The authors declare no conflict of interest.

References and Notes

1. Oikawa, M.; Hobo, S.; Oyamada, T.; Yoshikawa, H. Effects of orientation, intermittent rest and vehicle cleaning during transport on development of transport-related respiratory disease in horses. *J. Comp. Pathol.* **2005**, *132*, 153–168.

2. Salak-Johnson, J.; McGlone, J. Making sense of apparently conflicting data: Stress and immunity in swine and cattle. *J. Anim. Sci.* **2007**, *85*, E81–E88.

3. Fallani, G.; Prato Previde, E.; Valsecchi, P. Behavioral and physiological responses of guide dogs to a situation of emotional distress. *Physiol. Behav.* **2007**, *90*, 648–655.

4. Hiby, E.F.; Rooney, N.J.; Bradshaw, J.W.S. Behavioural and physiological responses of dogs entering re-homing kennels. *Physiol. Behav.* **2006**, *89*, 385–391.

5. King, T.; Hemsworth, P.H.; Coleman, G.J. Fear of novel and startling stimuli in domestic dogs. *Appl. Anim. Behav. Sci.* **2003**, *82*, 45–64.

6. Sales, G.; Hubrecht, R.; Peyvandi, A.; Milligan, S.; Shield, B. Noise in dog kennelling: Is barking a welfare problem for dogs? *Appl. Anim. Behav. Sci.* **1997**, *52*, 321–329.

7. Hubrecht, R.C.; Serpell, J.A.; Poole, T.B. Correlates of pen size and housing conditions on the behaviour of kennelled dogs. *Appl. Anim. Behav. Sci.* **1992**, *34*, 365–383.

8. Beerda, B.; Schilder, M.B.H.; Bernadina, W.; Van Hooff, J.A.R.A.M.; De Vries, H.W.; Mol, J.A. Chronic stress in dogs subjected to social and spatial restriction. II. Hormonal and immunological responses. *Physiol. Behav.* **1999**, *66*, 243–254.

9. Väisänen, M.A.-M.; Valros, A.E.; Hakaoja, E.; Raekallio, M.R.; Vainio, O.M. Pre-operative stress in dogs—A preliminary investigation of behavior and heart rate variability in healthy hospitalized dogs. *Vet. Anaesth. Analg.* **2005**, *32*, 158–167.

10. Ward, P.A.; Blanchard, R.J.; Bolivar, V.; Brown, M.J.; Chang, F.; Herman, J.P.; Zawistowski, S.L. *Recognition and Alleviation of Distress in Laboratory Animals*; National Academies Press: Washington, DC, USA, 2008.

11. Sapolsky, R.M.; Romero, L.M.; Munck, A.U. How do glucocorticoids influence stress responses? Integrating permissive, suppressive, stimulatory, and preparative actions. *Endocr. Rev.* **2000**, *21*, 55–89.

12. Romero, L.M.; Butler, L.K. Endocrinology of stress. *Int. J. Comp. Psychol.* **2007**, *20*, 89–95.

13. Remer, T.; Maser-Gluth, C.; Wudy, S. Glucocorticoid measurements in health and disease—Metabolic implications and the potential of 24-h urine analyses. *Mini Rev. Med. Chem.* **2008**, *8*, 153–170.

14. Wray, C.J.; Mammen, J.; Hasselgren, P.-O. Catabolic response to stress and potential benefits of nutrition support. *Nutrition* **2002**, *18*, 971–977.

15. Taché, Y.; Bonaz, B. Corticotropin-releasing factor receptors and stress-related alterations of gut motor function. *J. Clin. Invest.* **2007**, *117*, 33–40.

16. Bueno, L.; Fioramonti, J. Effects of corticotropin-releasing factor, corticotropin and cortisol on gastrointestinal motility in dogs. *Peptides* **1986**, *7*, 73–77.

17. Aoyagi, T.; Izumi, Y.; Hiroyama, M.; Matsuzaki, T.; Yasuoka, Y.; Sanbe, A.; Tanoue, A. Vasopressin regulates the renin-angiotensin-aldosterone system via V1a receptors in macula densa cells. *Am. J. Physiol. Renal Physiol.* **2008**, *295*, F100–F107.

18. Charmandari, E.; Tsigos, C.; Chrousos, G. Endocrinology of the stress response. *Annu. Rev. Physiol.* **2005**, *67*, 259–284.

19. Dhabhar, F.S. A hassle a day may keep the pathogens away: The fight-or-flight stress response and the augmentation of immune function. *Integr. Comp. Biol.* **2009**, *49*, 215–236.

20. Hänsel, A.; Hong, S.; Cámara, R.J.A.; Von Kaenel, R. Inflammation as a psychophysiological biomarker in chronic psychosocial stress. *Neurosci. Biobehav. Rev.* **2010**, *35*, 115–121.

21. Bellomo, R.; Ronco, C.; Kellum, J.A.; Mehta, R.L.; Palevsky, P.; Acute Dialysis Quality Initiative workgroup. Acute renal failure—Definition, outcome measures, animal models, fluid therapy and information technology needs: The Second International Consensus Conference of the Acute Dialysis Quality Initiative (ADQI) Group. *Crit. Care* **2004**, *8*, R204–R212.

22. Depke, M.; Steil, L.; Domanska, G.; Völker, U.; Schütt, C.; Kiank, C. Altered hepatic mRNA expression of immune response and apoptosis-associated genes after acute and chronic psychological stress in mice. *Mol. Immunol.* **2009**, *46*, 3018–3028.

23. Siracusa, C.; Manteca, X.; Cerón, J.; Martínez-Subiela, S.; Cuenca, R.; Lavín, S.; Garcia, F.; Pastor, J. Perioperative stress response in dogs undergoing elective surgery: Variations in behavioural, neuroendocrine, immune and acute phase responses. *Anim. Welf.* **2008**, *17*, 259–273.

24. Sgoifo, A.; Koolhaas, J.M.; Musso, E.; De Boer, S.F. Different Sympathovagal Modulation of Heart Rate During Social and Nonsocial Stress Episodes in Wild-Type Rats. *Physiol. Behav.* **1999**, *67*, 733–738.

25. Dess, N.K.; Linwick, D.; Patterson, J.; Overmier, J.B.; Levine, S. Immediate and proactive effects of controllability and predictability on plasma cortisol responses to shocks in dogs. *Behav. Neurosci.* **1983**, *97*, 1005–1016.

26. Bowers, S.L.; Bilbo, S.D.; Dhabhar, F.S.; Nelson, R.J. Stressor-specific alterations in corticosterone and immune responses in mice. *Brain. Behav. Immun.* **2008**, *22*, 105–113.

27. Dickerson, S.S.; Kemeny, M.E. Acute stressors and cortisol responses: A theoretical integration and synthesis of laboratory research. *Psychol. Bull.* **2004**, *130*, 355–391.

28. Glaser, R.; Kiecolt-Glaser, J.K. Stress-induced immune dysfunction: Implications for health. *Nat. Rev. Immunol.* **2005**, *5*, 243–251.

29. Royer, C.M.; Willard, M.; Williamson, K.; Steiner, J.M.; Williams, D.A.; Davis, M. Exercise stress, intestinal permeability and gastric ulceration in racing Alaskan sled dogs. *Equine Comp. Exerc. Physiol.* **2005**, *2*, 53–59.

30. Vitalo, A.; Fricchione, J.; Casali, M.; Berdichevsky, Y.; Hoge, E.A.; Rauch, S.L.; Berthiaume, F.; Yarmush, M.L.; Benson, H.; Fricchione, G.L.; Levine, J.B. Nest Making and Oxytocin Comparably Promote Wound Healing in Isolation Reared Rats. *PLoS ONE* **2009**, *4*, doi:10.1371/journal.pone.0005523.

31. Dreschel, N.A. The effects of fear and anxiety on health and lifespan in pet dogs. *Appl. Anim. Behav. Sci.* **2010**, *125*, 157–162.

32. Segerstrom, S.C.; Miller, G.E. Psychological stress and the human immune system: A meta-analytic study of 30 years of inquiry. *Psychol. Bull.* **2004**, *130*, 601–630.

33. Elenkov, I.J. Glucocorticoids and the Th1/Th2 balance. *Ann. N. Y. Acad. Sci.* **2004**, *1024*, 138–146.

34. Palsgaard-Van Lue, A.; Jensen, A.L.; Strøm, H.; Kristensen, A.T. Comparative analysis of haematological, haemostatic, and inflammatory parameters in canine venous and arterial blood samples. *Vet. J.* **2007**, *173*, 664–668.

35. Engler, H.; Dawils, L.; Hoves, S.; Kurth, S.; Stevenson, J.R.; Schauenstein, K.; Stefanski, V. Effects of social stress on blood leukocyte distribution: The role of alpha- and beta-adrenergic mechanisms. *J. Neuroimmunol.* **2004**, *156*, 153–162.

36. Steptoe, A.; Hamer, M.; Chida, Y. The effects of acute psychological stress on circulating inflammatory factors in humans: A review and meta-analysis. *Brain. Behav. Immun.* **2007**, *21*, 901–912.

37. Kiank, C.; Holtfreter, B.; Starke, A.; Mundt, A.; Wilke, C.; Schutt, C.; Heijnen, C.; Kavelaars, A.; Schütt, C. Stress susceptibility predicts the severity of immune depression and the failure to combat bacterial infections in chronically stressed mice. *Brain. Behav. Immun.* **2006**, *20*, 359–368.

38. Kiank, C.; Entleutner, M.; Fürll, B.; Westerholt, A.; Heidecke, C.-D.D.; Schütt, C. Stress-induced immune conditioning affects the course of experimental peritonitis. *Shock* **2007**, *27*, 305–311.

39. Webster Marketon, J.I.; Glaser, R. Stress hormones and immune function. *Cell. Immunol.* **2008**, *252*, 16–26.

40. Avitsur, R.; Powell, N.; Padgett, D.; Sheridan, J. Social interactions, stress, and immunity. *Immunol. Allergy Clin. North Am.* **2009**, *29*, 285–293.

41. Dhabhar, S.; Viswanathan, K. Short-term stress experienced at time of immunization induces a long-lasting increase in immunologic memory. *Am. J. Physiol. Regul. Integr. Comp. Physiol.* **2005**, *289*, R738–R744.

42. Viswanathan, K.; Daugherty, C.; Dhabhar, F.S. Stress as an endogenous adjuvant: Augmentation of the immunization phase of cell-mediated immunity. *Inter. Immunol.* **2005**, *17*, 1059–1069.

43. Miller, G.E. Psychological stress and antibody response to influenza vaccination: When is the critical period for stress, and how does it get inside the body? *Psychosom. Med.* **2004**, *66*, 215–223.

44. Otto, C.M. Sepsis in veterinary patients: What do we know and where can we go? *J. Vet. Emerg. Crit. Care* **2007**, *17*, 329–332.

45. Broadbent, E. Psychological Stress Impairs Early Wound Repair Following Surgery. *Psychosom. Med.* **2003**, *65*, 865–869.

46. Vileikyte, L. Stress and wound healing. *Clin. Dermatol.* **2007**, *25*, 49–55.

47. Caso, J.R.; Leza, J.C.; Menchen, L.; Menchén, L. The effects of physical and psychological stress on the gastro-intestinal tract: Lessons from animal models. *Curr. Mol. Med.* **2008**, *8*, 299–312.

48. Maunder, R.; Levenstein, S. The Role of Stress in the Development and Clinical Course of Inflammatory Bowel Disease: Epidemiological Evidence. *Curr. Mol. Med.* **2008**, *8*, 247–252.

49. Leib, M.S. Treatment of Chronic Idiopathic Large-Bowel Diarrhea in Dogs with a Highly Digestible Diet and Soluble Fiber: A Retrospective Review of 37 Cases. *J. Vet. Int. Med.* **2000**, *14*, 27–32.

50. Davis, M.S.; Willard, M.D.; Nelson, S.L.; Mandsager, R.E.; McKiernan, B.S.; Mansell, J.K.; Lehenbauer, T.W. Prevalence of Gastric Lesions in Racing Alaskan Sled Dogs. *J. Vet. Intern. Med.* **2003**, *17*, 311–314.

51. Kovach, J.A.; Nearing, B.D.; Verrier, R.L. Angerlike behavioral state potentiates myocardial ischemia-induced T-wave alternans in canines. *J. Am. Coll. Cardiol.* **2001**, *37*, 1719–1725.

52. Ziegelstein, R.C. Acute emotional stress and cardiac arrhythmias. *JAMA* **2007**, *298*, 324–329.

53. Von Känel, R.; Dimsdale, J.E.; Patterson, T.L.; Grant, I.; Känel, R. Acute procoagulant stress response as a dynamic measure of allostatic load in Alzheimer caregivers. *Ann. Behav. Med.* **2003**, *26*, 42–48.

54. Wirtz, P.H.; Redwine, L.S.; Baertschi, C.; Spillmann, M.; Ehlert, U.; von Känel, R. Coagulation activity before and after acute psychosocial stress increases with age. *Psychosom. Med.* **2008**, *70*, 476–481.

55. Dimsdale, J.E. Psychological Stress and Cardiovascular Disease. *J. Am. Coll. Cardiol.* **2008**, *51*, 1237–1246.

56. Esler, M.; Eikelis, N.; Schlaich, M.; Lambert, G.; Alvarenga, M.; Dawood, T.; Kaye, D.; Barton, D.; Pier, C.; Guo, L.; Brenchley, C.; Jennings, G.; Lambert, E. Chronic mental stress is a cause of essential hypertension: Presence of biological markers of stress. *Clin. Exp. Pharmacol. Physiol.* **2008**, *35*, 498–502.

57. Hamer, M.; O'Donnell, K.; Lahiri, A.; Steptoe, A. Salivary cortisol responses to mental stress are associated with coronary artery calcification in healthy men and women. *Eur. Heart J.* **2010**, *31*, 424–429.

58. Haverbeke, A.; Diederich, C.; Depiereux, E.; Giffroy, J.M. Cortisol and behavioral responses of working dogs to environmental challenges. *Physiol. Behav.* **2008**, *93*, 59–67.

59. Hellhammer, D.H.; Wüst, S.; Kudielka, B.M. Salivary cortisol as a biomarker in stress research. *Psychoneuroendocrinology* **2009**, *34*, 163–171.

60. Rooney, N.J.; Gaines, S.A.; Bradshaw, J.W.S. Behavioural and glucocorticoid responses of dogs (*Canis familiaris*) to kennelling: Investigating mitigation of stress by prior habituation. *Physiol. Behav.* **2007**, *92*, 847–854.

61. Vincent, I.C.; Michell, A.R. Comparison of cortisol concentrations in saliva and plasma of dogs. *Res. Vet. Sci.* **1992**, *53*, 342–345.

62. Kobelt, A.J.; Hemsworth, P.H.; Barnett, J.L.; Butler, K.L. Sources of sampling variation in saliva cortisol in dogs. *Res. Vet. Sci.* **2003**, *75*, 157–161.

63. Levine, A.; Zagoory-Sharon, O.; Feldman, R.; Lewis, J.G.; Weller, A. Measuring cortisol in human psychobiological studies. *Physiol. Behav.* **2007**, *90*, 43–53.

64. Schatz, S.; Palme, R. Measurement of Faecal Cortisol Metabolites in Cats and Dogs: A Non-invasive Method for Evaluating Adrenocortical Function. *Vet. Res. Commun.* **2001**, *25*, 271–287.

65. Hennessy, M.B. Using hypothalamic–pituitary–adrenal measures for assessing and reducing the stress of dogs in shelters: A review. *Appl. Anim. Behav. Sci.* **2013**, *149*, 1–12.

66. Ottenheimer Carrier, L.; Cyr, A.; Anderson, R.E.; Walsh, C.J. Exploring the dog park: Relationships between social behaviours, personality and cortisol in companion dogs. *Appl. Anim. Behav. Sci.* **2013**, *146*, 96–106.

67. Angle, C.T.; Wakshlag, J.J.; Gillette, R.L.; Stokol, T.; Geske, S.; Adkins, T.O.; Gregor, C. Hematologic, serum biochemical, and cortisol changes associated with anticipation of exercise and short duration high intensity exercise in sled dogs. *Vet. Clin. Pathol.* **2009**, *38*, 370–374.

68. Palme, R.; Rettenbacher, S.; Touma, C.; El-Bahr, S.M.; Möstl, E. Stress hormones in mammals and birds: Comparative aspects regarding metabolism, excretion, and noninvasive measurement in fecal samples. *Ann. N. Y. Acad. Sci.* **2005**, *1040*, 162–171.

69. Kolevska, J.; Brunclik, V.; Svoboda, M. Circadian rhythm of cortisol secretion in dogs of different daily activities. *Acta Vet. Brno* **2003**, *72*, 599–605.

70. Durocher, L.L.; Hinchcliff, K.W.; Williamson, K.K.; McKenzie, E.C.; Holbrook, T.C.; Willard, M.; Royer, C.M.; Davis, M.S. Effect of strenuous exercise on urine concentrations of homovanillic acid, cortisol, and vanillylmandelic acid in sled dogs. *Am. J. Vet. Res.* **2007**, *68*, 107–111.

71. Raekallio, M.R.; Kuusela, E.K.; Lehtinen, M.E.; Tykkyloinen, M.K.; Huttunen, P.; Westerholm, F.C. Effects of exercise-induced stress and dexamethasone on plasma hormone and glucose concentrations and sedation in dogs treated with dexmedetomidine. *Am. J. Vet. Res.* **2005**, *66*, 260–265.

72. Takahashi, A.; Uchiyama, S.; Kato, Y. Immunochromatographic assay using gold nanoparticles for measuring salivary secretory IgA in dogs as a stress marker. *Sci. Technol. Adv. Mater.* **2009**, *10*, doi:10.1088/1468-6996/10/3/034604.

73. Kikkawa, A.; Uchida, Y.; Nakade, T.; Taguchi, K. Salivary secretory IgA concentrations in beagle dogs. *J. Vet. Med. Sci.* **2003**, *65*, 689–693.

74. Skandakumar, S.; Stodulski, G.; Hau, J. Salivary IgA: A possible stress marker in dogs. *Anim. Welf.* **1995**, *4*, 339–350.

75. Takahashi, I.; Nochi, T.; Kunisawa, J. The mucosal immune system for secretory IgA responses and mucosal vaccine development. *Inflamm. Regen.* **2010**, *30*, 40–47.

76. Davis, A.K.; Maney, D.L.; Maerz, J.C. The use of leukocyte profiles to measure stress in vertebrates: A review for ecologists. *Funct. Ecol.* **2008**, *22*, 760–772.

77. Beerda, B.; Schilder, M.B.H.; van Hooff, J.A.R.A.M.; de Vries, H.W.; Mol, J.A. Behavioural, saliva cortisol and heart rate responses to different types of stimuli in dogs. *Appl. Anim. Behav. Sci.* **1998**, *58*, 365–381.

78. Palestrini, C.; Previde, E.P.; Spiezio, C.; Verga, M. Heart rate and behavioural responses of dogs in the Ainsworth's Strange Situation: A pilot study. *Appl. Anim. Behav. Sci.* **2005**, *94*, 75–88.

79. Maros, K.; Dóka, A.; Miklósi, Á. Behavioural correlation of heart rate changes in family dogs. *Appl. Anim. Behav. Sci.* **2008**, *109*, 329–341.

80. Wang, X.; Ding, X.; Su, S.; Li, Z.; Riese, H.; Thayer, J.F.; Treiber, F.; Snieder, H. Genetic influences on heart rate variability at rest and during stress. *Psychophysiology* **2009**, *46*, 458–465.

81. Jonckheer-Sheehy, V.S.M.; Vinke, C.M.; Ortolani, A. Validation of a Polar® human heart rate monitor for measuring heart rate and heart rate variability in adult dogs under stationary conditions. *J. Vet. Behav. Clin. Appl. Res.* **2012**, *7*, 205–212.

82. Essner, A.; Sjöström, R.; Ahlgren, E.; Lindmark, B. Validity and reliability of Polar® RS800CX heart rate monitor, measuring heart rate in dogs during standing position and at trot on a treadmill. *Physiol. Behav.* **2013**, *114*, 1–5.

83. Engeland, W.C.; Miller, P.; Gann, D.S. Pituitary-adrenal adrenomedullary responses to noise in awake dogs. *Am. J. Physiol.* **1990**, *258*, R672–R677.

84. Kudielka, B.M.; Buske-Kirschbaum, A.; Hellhammer, D.H.; Kirschbaum, C. HPA axis responses to laboratory psychosocial stress in healthy elderly adults, younger adults, and children: Impact of age and gender. *Psychoneuroendocrinology* **2004**, *29*, 83–98.

85. Beerda, B.; Schilder, M.B.H.; van Hooff, J.A.R.A.M.; de Vries, H.W.; Mol, J.A. Behavioural and hormonal indicators of enduring environmental stress in dogs. *Anim. Welf.* **2000**, *9*, 49–62.

86. Holton, L.; Pawson, P.; Nolan, A.; Reid, J.; Scott, E.M. Development of a behaviour-based scale to measure acute pain in dogs. *Vet. Rec.* **2001**, *148*, 525–531.

87. Hudson, J.T.; Slater, M.R.; Taylor, L.; Scott, H.M.; Kerwin, S.C. Assessing repeatability and validity of a visual analogue scale questionnaire for use in assessing pain and lameness in dogs. *Am. J. Vet. Res.* **2004**, *65*, 1634–1643.

88. Morton, C.M.; Reid, J.; Scott, E.M.; Holton, L.L.; Nolan, A.M. Application of a scaling model to establish and validate an interval level pain scale for assessment of acute pain in dogs. *Am. J. Vet. Res.* **2005**, *66*, 2154–2166.

89. Hekman, J.P.; Karas, A.Z.; Dreschel, N.A. Salivary cortisol concentrations and behavior in a population of healthy dogs hospitalized for elective procedures. *Appl. Anim. Behav. Sci.* **2012**, *141*, 149–157.

3

Social Networks and Welfare in Future Animal Management

Paul Koene [1,*] **and Bert Ipema** [2]

[1] Department of Animal Welfare, Wageningen UR Livestock Research, P.O. Box 65, 8200 AB Lelystad, The Netherlands

[2] Department of Farm Systems, Wageningen UR Livestock Research, P.O. Box 65, 8200 AB Lelystad, The Netherlands; E-Mail: bert.ipema@wur.nl

* Author to whom correspondence should be addressed; E-Mail: paul.koene@wur.nl.

Simple Summary: Living in a stable social environment is important to animals. Animal species have developed social behaviors and rules of approach and avoidance of conspecifics in order to co-exist. Animal species are kept or domesticated without explicit regard for their inherent social behavior and rules. Examples of social structures are provided for four species kept and managed by humans. This information is important for the welfare management of these species. In the near future, automatic measurement of social structures will provide a tool for daily welfare management together with nearest neighbor information.

Abstract: It may become advantageous to keep human-managed animals in the social network groups to which they have adapted. Data concerning the social networks of farm animal species and their ancestors are scarce but essential to establishing the importance of a natural social network for farmed animal species. Social Network Analysis (SNA) facilitates the characterization of social networking at group, subgroup and individual levels. SNA is currently used for modeling the social behavior and management of wild animals and social welfare of zoo animals. It has been recognized for use with farm animals but has yet to be applied for management purposes. Currently, the main focus is on cattle, because in large groups (poultry), recording of individuals is expensive and the existence of social networks is uncertain due to on-farm restrictions. However, in many cases, a stable social network might be important to individual animal fitness, survival and welfare. For instance, when laying hens are not too densely housed, simple networks may be established. We describe here small social networks in horses, brown bears, laying hens and veal calves to illustrate the importance of measuring social networks among animals managed by humans. Emphasis is placed on the automatic measurement of identity, location, nearest neighbors and nearest neighbor distance for management purposes. It is concluded that social networks are important to the welfare of human-managed animal species and that welfare management based on automatic recordings will become available in the near future.

Keywords: Social Network Analysis; SNA; captive animals; animal management; approach-avoidance behavior; animal welfare; *Ursus arctos*; *Equus caballus*; *Gallus gallus domesticus*; *Bos taurus*

1. General Introduction

Hale [1] proposed that certain wild animal characteristics favored domestication. Indeed, domestic animals tend to be large, non-selective feeders that occupy open habitats. They are socially organized non-territorial species, typically occurring in relatively large groups in their natural environments. There are pros and cons to the grouping of animals. A strong social network is required to maintain the group and to allow them to cope with environmental challenges. In captivity, such networks may or may not exist, depending on actual group size and living conditions. In terms of evolution, it may be advantageous to keep animals in the groups to which they have become accustomed [2]. Data concerning social networks under farm animal species is scarce but is essential for the establishment of the importance of such networks. Additionally, deviations within a social network, such as an individual that gradually disassociates itself from the network, may provide essential information concerning health or welfare.

Social Network Analysis (SNA) facilitates the characterization of network behavior and preferences at group, subgroup and individual levels. The study of animal social networks has become increasingly popular in many areas of behavioral research [3–5] and the temporal aspects of networks attract attention [6]; linking both individual behavior to population patterns and *vice versa* [7] to and personality [8]. Technical advances will make it possible to analyze whole populations in the near future [9–11]. Epidemiologists use SNA to model disease transfer and probably to understand the spreading of behavioral problems (*i.e.*, feather pecking in laying hens [12,13]). Application of SNA has improved our understanding of animal welfare in Atlantic salmons [14], rhesus macaques [15], pigtailed macaques [16], giraffes [17,18] and African elephants [19]. Knowledge concerning important or detrimental animals in the network forms a basis for management actions, such as removal of individuals from the group [5,16,20]. Removal of certain pigtailed macaques (*Macaca nemestrina*) resulted in decreased grooming, increased aggression and influenced the network structure [16].

Currently, social networks are often investigated for several reasons, one of which is the determination of animal social welfare [12–14,16,21]. Stable and suitable relationships support the social network and its individuals (social support [22–24]), while unstable and unsuitable networks may generate social stress [25–27]. In many cases, as with broilers or laying hens, groups are so large that nearest neighbors are probably strangers, casting doubt on the existence of a real social network and individual recognition. However, in many cases social networks might be important to animal fitness, survival and welfare [28,29]. Mismatches that have evolved within a species' social network and the actual social network in a managed housing system should be observed and recorded [28]. Individual animals can react to correct mismatches, *i.e.*, approach or seek other animals or commodities (preferred) or flee to avoid other animals or commodities (non-preferred).

Network analysis can reveal positive (individuals approach each other; social support; approaching) or negative (individuals avoid each other; social stress; avoiding) associations between individual animals (Mode-1 networks) or between individual animals and their environment (food, cover) or events (aggression, predation) in so-called "affiliation networks" (Mode-2 networks). Social networks describe and analyze the positive and negative associations between individuals. Conflicts between approach and avoidance tendencies in individuals may compromise animal welfare when not quickly and adequately resolved [30–32]. This may well be due to those animals displaying neither significant approach (towards neighbors) nor avoidance (of conspecifics) in the social network.

We present some examples and data of small social networks in horses, brown bears, chicken and veal calves. In these four examples (#1–#4) social behavior, welfare and management are relevant. Simple management advice about removal (example#1—horses), management in large enclosures (example#2—brown bears), feather pecking (example#3—laying hens) and social housing (example#4—veal calves) are given. The four species are described to illustrate the social networks of social and solitary species in wild, semi-wild and domesticated conditions, under extensive or intensive management. The species were observed using various observation methods (nearest neighbor, x-y coordinates, visual, video and automated recording). Based on these differences, some hypotheses were formulated. Comparison of the examples may shed some light on differences in social networks of presumed solitary and social species, on space use and on the use of certain observation methods. Some general hypotheses have been formulated that will be elaborated further in the general discussion. The hypotheses are: (1) Solitary species have lower density networks than social species, (2) measurement of proximity (*i.e.*, nearest neighbors and/or nearest neighbor distances) is enough and supported with location measurements, (3) automated measurement of locations allows for quick measurement of nearest neighbor (NN), nearest neighbor distance (NND), locations, location of facilities and, consequently, changes in social networks can be determined on-line.

Nearest neighbor matrices can be made for each species, analyzed in a standard way using MatMan™ [33], UciNet [34] and NetDraw [35]. An example of nearest neighbor validation measurements using behavior observations in the horse is shown (Table 1). Further emphasis is placed on the importance of location for interpretation of nearest neighbor information in brown bears and laying hens and automatic measurement of location and/or nearest neighbors for management purposes using data on veal calves (Table 1). It is concluded that social networks are important to the welfare of captive animal species, and in the near future knowledge of social behavior and automatic recording will facilitate management.

Table 1. Overview of the presented Social Networks based on nearest neighbors of animals.

Example	#1	#2	#3	#4
Species	Equus caballus	Ursus arctos	Gallus gallus domesticus	Bos taurus
Example	Mares and foals	Dancing bears	Laying hens	Veal calves
Environment	Free range	Large bear enclosure	Stable	Stable
NN-measurement	Observer in the field	Observer in zoo	Video observations	Location sensors
Social life	Social	Solitary	Small groups, solitary	Social
SNA	1-mode	1-mode	1-mode, 2-mode	1-mode, 2-mode

2. General Methods—SNA

A social network consists of a number of nodes (individuals) and edges (relations between two nodes or individuals) [13]. Many concepts and parameters are developed to characterize and compare each node, detect relevant node subgroups within a network and characterize the network as a whole [36]. Basic input of Social Network Analysis (SNA) are associations between individuals; in this paper nearest neighbors associations or pairs are measured.

Data of nearest neighbor pairs (X-Y coordinates or recording nearest neighbors) was collected using scan sampling. Data is selected from the daylight period in which all four species are the most active, although night activity in horses and bears is possible.

Associations between individuals were calculated initially using the simple ratio index [37] (frequency of being nearest neighbor divided by the total number of observations), but here the nearest neighbor (NN)-matrix was used, because all animals remained visible in every observation and thus the outcomes of both methods were the same. Preferred associations are nearest neighbor pairs that are observed (o) significantly more often than expected (e) according to the standardized residual ($SR = (o-e)/\sqrt{e}$), while pairs that avoid each other are observed less frequently than expected. The standardized residuals were calculated in MatMan™ [33]. These residuals showed significance at a P-value < 0.05 with standardized residuals of ≥ 1.96 and ≤ -1.96 [38]. Two matrices were constructed: (a) a positive matrix, in which positive significant associations (positive SR > 1.96) were determined with other values (SR < 1.96) set at zero and (b) a negative matrix in which negative significant associations (SR < -1.96) were determined (and made positive by multiplying SR by -1) with other values (SR > -1.96) set at zero. Both matrices provided weighted input for UciNet [34]. The resulting UciNet data file supplied input for UciNet or NetDraw [35] procedures. The resulting data can be interpreted in several ways (Table 2).

Table 2. Possible interpretations of nearest neighbor data from nearest neighbor matrices.

Standardized Residuals (SR)	>1.96	<−1.96
Social Network	Positive	Negative
Preference	Affection	Aversion
Motivation	Approach/seek	Avoidance/escape
Social behavior	Socio-positive (support?)	Socio-negative (stress?)
Individual welfare	Positive?	Negative?

The four animal species were monitored on a number of subsequent or consecutive days. Some parameters of SNA were calculated or visualized in NetDraw and UciNet: nodes (components of a network with known relationships, here individual animals), edges (also line or tie, is a relationship between two nodes of a network; strength is shown by line thickness) and resulting graphs (a set of nodes and edges, visualized as a picture showing dots connected by lines; labels in the graph are placed to the right of the nodes/individuals, thickness of the lines relative to SR-value). Arrows on the lines are directed, *i.e.*, the focal animal and/or nearest neighbor of the focal animal are indicated. Lines with two arrows indicate a bidirectional relationship (two-way); lines with a single arrow a unidirectional (one-way) relationship. A graph based on significant positive associations indicates a positive network; a graph based on significant negative associations indicates a negative network. Graphs are characterized by the group measure of density (calculated in UciNet; the proportion of all possible connections that are significant for the positive network (SR > 1.96) and for the negative network (SR < −1.96); the more significant the relationships, the higher the density.

The importance of the nodes (individuals) is often characterized by degree of centrality, betweenness centrality and closeness centrality [39,40]. Degree (number of connections a focal animal has with other group members), betweenness (the number of shortest paths between every pair of other group members on which the focal individual lies) and closeness (closeness is defined as the inverse of the farness; farness is defined as the sum of its distances to all other group members) are shown in the tables. In addition, subgroup information is given in the tables by cutpoints (which locate parts of the social network that would become disconnected if either an individual or connection were removed) and blocks (which are the resulting subgroups of individuals; the cutpoint is the individual that would, if removed, create the disconnection). Cutpoint and block presence (1) or absence (0) are given per individual. Cutpoints are biologically important individuals that should be removed to prevent disease transfer or that should not be removed to maintain the social network. Averages of node degree, betweenness, closeness, cutpoints and blocks are given in the tables; average cutpoint and block represent the proportion of individuals who are a cutpoint or part of a block. Data presented in this paper is output from NetDraw (within UciNet); from the *analysis* menu *centrality measures* and *blocks & cutpoints* have been activated; data from the *node attribute editor* was copied; NetDraw labels *farness* wrongly as *closeness*). Only undirected relationships are shown in the tables.

It is important for animals in a group to have stable and predictable relations with other animals in the group. The stability of a group is measured using the day-to-day variation of nearest neighbor relations in the group. The stability of the networks is thus given by the correlations between subsequent (and often consecutive) daily nearest neighbor matrices, calculated with the Mantel-test available in MatMan™ [33]. Significantly positive correlations imply network stability.

In addition to the social (1-mode) network, a 2-mode affiliation network (network exploring relationships between entities and events [12]) is given to show positive and negative significant individual-facility/commodity associations. In bipartite graphs for laying hens and veal calves examples are given of the positive or negative associations between individuals and facilities/commodities such as food, cubicles and nesting box. NetDraw provides graphs for these sub-structures and saves the information in the node attribute database.

In the general discussion the networks determined for the four example species are compared using network densities. Additionally, the percentage of density in the positive network—compared with total density—provides a characterization of both the positive and negative networks. An indication of network stability is provided by the average of the day-to-day correlations of nearest neighbor matrices.

3. Example#1: Outdoor Horses—Direct Observation of Location

Much research has been performed on the social interactions and relationships between horses [41]. Age and order of arrival in the group are important determinants of rank. Within herds, horses often form stronger social affiliations with animals from similar social or age classes. Such peer attachments can last for several years during which the bond between mares appears stronger than between bachelor stallions. These strong long-term affiliations between mares contribute greatly to the stability of the herd. Affiliated animals participate in social activities such as mutual grooming and play and tolerate each other in close proximity [41,42]. Despite this knowledge on individual relationships, not much is known about the composition of the social network and existing bonds between horses. Other *equid* species have been the subject of SNA [43]. The lack of publications on SNA in the domestic horse (*Equus caballus*) is remarkable, despite the obvious potential for SNA [44]. We recorded nearest neighbors in horses in order to understand their social network to facilitate management of mare-foal relations. Some specific hypotheses were formulated. The lone dam (Mare2) has no relations with the foals. Foal1 is 3 yrs. of age and will be removed from the group; she is expected to have relations with the dams and few relations with the other foals.

3.1. Materials and Methods

Social networks of Dartmoor ponies were studied in 2011. The ponies, owned by Unifarm of Wageningen University, were kept at pasture at the Organic Experimental and Training Farm "Droevendaal", the Netherlands. The herd under observation was kept outdoors under semi-feral conditions on an extensively managed pasture. The herd of mares comprised animals of different ages. The adult mares had been together in the Droevendaal herd since 2005. There were four dam/foal couples (mare and foal pairs that have the same numeric identifier) of which one was still nursing (Mare5-Foal5). Mare2 had no foal. The foals are of different ages Foal1 (3 yr.), Foal3 and Foal4 (2 yr.) and Foal5 (1 yr). An area of 4.35 ha extensively managed grassland was divided into 20 × 20 m plots (by numbered pavement tiles) to facilitate determination of the relative position of the ponies on the pasture. All animals were observed using continuous behavioral and simultaneous scan sampling. During continuous behavioral sampling, the social interactions "allogrooming" and "agonistic behavior" were recorded for a period of 50 hours. The location of the horse was recorded on paper with an image of the 20 × 20 m grid structure in the pasture. Coordinates (X-Y) were determined using scanned images of the mapped data and DataThief [45]. Nearest neighbors were determined using SpPack [46]. The method of analysis for the resulting NN-matrix is described in General methods—Paragraph 2. In order to determine a realistic image of the social network, the herd was observed for 8 days (*i.e.*, 440 scans per animal) during July 2011. In a subsequent study, the stability of the network was investigated further by daily removals of individual horses [47].

3.2. Results and Discussion

The average NND was 8.78 meter (SD of 8.98 meters). The network based on positive associations has a density of 0.21 and shows strong associations between Mare1-Foal1, Mare4-Foal4 and Mare5-Foal5 (Figure 1; left graph). Pair Mare3-Foal3 displays no significant relationship, but Mare2, Mare3 and Mare4 do. Foal4 has the most associations. The negative network, (Figure 1; right graph) density 0.31, shows that unrelated mares and foals avoid each other, while foals do not avoid each other and that Mare5 is often avoided. The strongest negative association is between Mare2 and Foal4 (thickest line).

Figure 1. Social networks of Dartmoor ponies on extensive pasture, based on significant positive associations (left graph) and negative associations (right graph). Note that some individual attributes (mare/foal and their genetic relation) are given.

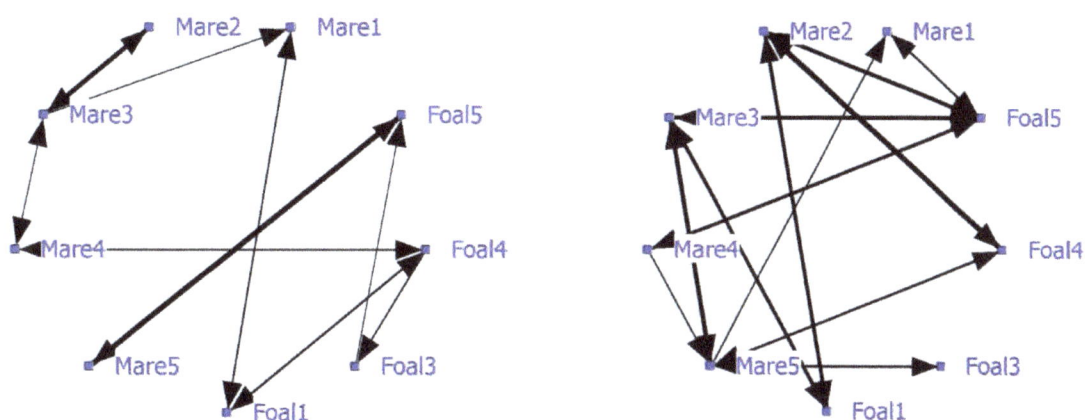

Foal4 has the highest node degree, a higher betweenness and lower farness than the other foals (Table 3). Mare2 and Mare5 have few significant connections, low betweenness and a high farness; they are relatively isolated from the rest. Based on two cutpoints (Mare3 and Foal5) three subgroups are distinguished: Block1 (Mare2 and Mare3), Block2 (Mare5 and Foal5) and Block3, a rest group connected by Mare3 and Foal5.

Table 3. Social Network Analysis (SNA) characteristics for individual and subgroup characteristics of Dartmoor ponies in an extensive pasture.

ID	Degree	Betweenness	Farness	Cutpoint	Block 1	Block 2	Block 3
Foal1	2	4	27	0	0	0	1
Foal3	2	12	27	0	0	0	1
Foal4	3	16	24	0	0	0	1
Foal5	2	7	32	1	0	1	1
Mare1	2	2	29	0	0	0	1
Mare2	1	0	35	0	1	0	0
Mare3	3	8	28	1	1	0	1
Mare4	2	8	26	0	0	0	1
Mare5	1	0	39	0	0	1	0
Average	2.00	6.33	29.67	0.22	0.22	0.22	0.78

For cutpoint and blocks: 0 = no and 1 = yes

The stability of the positive social network is shown by the positive significant correlations between NN-matrices on subsequent days and between 1 and 8 (Table 4).

Table 4. Nearest neighbor (NN)-Matrix correlations of eight consecutive days in Dartmoor ponies.

Days	1~2	2~3	3~4	4~5	5~6	6~7	7~8	1~8
Pearson's r	0.71	0.48	0.27	0.41	0.55	0.65	0.74	0.71
P-value	*0.001*	*0.003*	*0.049*	*0.008*	*0.002*	*0.001*	*0.001*	*0.001*

Between-horse social interaction was also observed to provide a matrix of grooming and agonistic interactions. Social grooming and agonistic interactions were not related (R = −0.05, P = 0.644). The observed social grooming interactions correlated significantly with NN-matrix (R = 0.70, P = 0.000); agonistic interactions did not (R = 0.16, P = 0.077). The NN-matrix indicates that subjects that are close together show allogrooming and positive social behavior. When horses allogroom, a reduction in heart rate is observed which may indicate social support [48] and positive welfare.

3.3. Management

We were able to determine social networks based on nearest neighbor data for an all mare herd of nine horses. All animals had one or more preferred companions, and relationships were typically between kin or peers. The network consisted of three subgroups: a basic group of mares and foals, a pair of two adult mares and one mare-foal pair with the foal still sucking. Grooming frequency was found to be significantly positively correlated with this social network, which validates use of proximity measures to analyze social affiliation in this particular group. This relationship needs to be verified for different/other groups, populations and species. Aggressive interactions did not correlate significantly within the network.

Foals were often sold at a young age. Foal1 (3 yr.) would be removed from the group, but still had significant positive relations with her mother and Foal4, and negative relations with Mare2 and Mare3. These findings are contrary to our expectations and hypothesis. On the other hand, Foal3 (2 yr.) no longer displayed a significant bond with her dam (Mare3) and showed only tentative dependencies with Foal4 and Foal5 and a socio-negative relationship with Mare5. Although Foal3 had a high betweenness, it was not a cutpoint and no separation issue was indicated, *i.e.*, removal had no influence on the subgroup structure. Based on these findings, it may be advisable to remove Foal3 instead of Foal1 from the group. The other foals maintained strong socio-positive bonds with their mothers, and removal of these foals presented a higher risk to the social structure and welfare of the group.

4. Example#2: Outdoor Brown Bears—Direct Observation of Location

Brown bears (*Ursus arctos*) are solitary animals except during breeding and cub rearing. In case of surplus food availability—salmon in rivers—large groups develop and a simple social organization develops [49,50]. Individuals typically have home ranges of 500–1500 square kilometers (males) and 100–800 square kilometers (females). Despite the fact that brown bears are territorial, their home ranges overlap, and boundaries are often not defended. In captivity brown bears are mostly kept in enclosures of a minimum of 400 m^2 and bears seem to be non-territorial. Recently, large bear enclosures (LBE) have become popular, demanding more from zookeepers and management, *i.e.*, electric fencing, feeding, environmental and veterinary management. Some scientific research has been done in LBEs and is helpful in feeding and social management of bears [51–53]. The social interactions between brown bears have been studied [52] and may play an important role in the positive social network [53]. In large bear enclosures (LBE) many brown bears can be housed, and these supposedly solitary animals are forced to develop social contacts, especially in feeding situations. There is a lack of knowledge about the social network in such situations. One of the hypotheses investigated is that brown bears have no territories in LBEs.

4.1. Material & Methods

In 1995 detailed positions and behaviors were registered for 15 individual bears in a 2-ha bear forest at Rhenen in the Netherlands. These brown bears were of different ages and sexes (all neutered). They had been rescued from dancing shows, restaurants or inadequate zoos. Bear08, Bear09 and Bear10 came as former dancing bears from Turkey and were blind. The activities, locations and nearest neighbors (NN) of these brown bears were recorded by volunteers in a 10-day period under strict pre-programmed conditions using check sheets and maps on which data of behavior and location were recorded. Maps were digitized and x-y coordinates of locations recorded using DataThief [45] and nearest neighbors were determined using SpPack [46]. Subsequent analysis of the NN-matrix is described in Paragraph 2 (general methods).

4.2. Results and Discussion

Significant positive associations were determined between some bears. The positive network showed a density of 0.16. The density of the negative network was 0.37 and was much higher than the density of the positive network. Nearest neighbor distances in the unlimited NN-matrix ranged from zero to 72 meter with an average of 13.36 meter (SD = 13.75 meters). Many individual bears appeared to have relatively fixed locations that may be territories or restricted home ranges and influence the associations and the network analysis. For instance, the blind Turkish bears (08, 09 and 10) occupied small areas that they hardly left. In a follow-up analysis, only nearest neighbors at a maximum NND of 5 meters were used (use of handmade notes on paper maps make a lower limit unreliable). Only 18% (638 of the 4710) of the NN-pair observations were used and the average NND was 3.38 meters (SD = 1.19 meter). The densities of the positive and negative network were 0.12 and 0.095, respectively. The correlation between the network using the NN-matrix with unlimited NND (N = 3491) and the network using max NND of 5 meters (N = 637) is 0.75 (P < 0.0001). The NND-limited network is shown in this paper (Figure 2). Bear02 and Bear03 were the only animals without any positive associations (solitary). Bears11, 12, 13 and 14 formed a pair-wise connected subgroup in the positive network (Figure 2; left graph; see also Table 5; Block 3, 4, 5) of young bears that roamed around with no fixed place in the enclosure. Furthermore, some strong pair associations (e.g., Bear04 and Bear05, Bear06 and Bear07, Bear01 and Bear09) were found. Bear09 and Bear10 were associated with Bear04. Negative associations were also found in the negative network (Figure 2; right graph). Six bears lacked negative associations while four bears had at least three negative associations (Bear04, Bear05, Bear12 and Bear13).

Figure 2. Social network of bears in a large bear enclosures (LBE) using a nearest neighbor distance (NND) smaller than 5 meter (positive network in left graph and negative network in right graph).

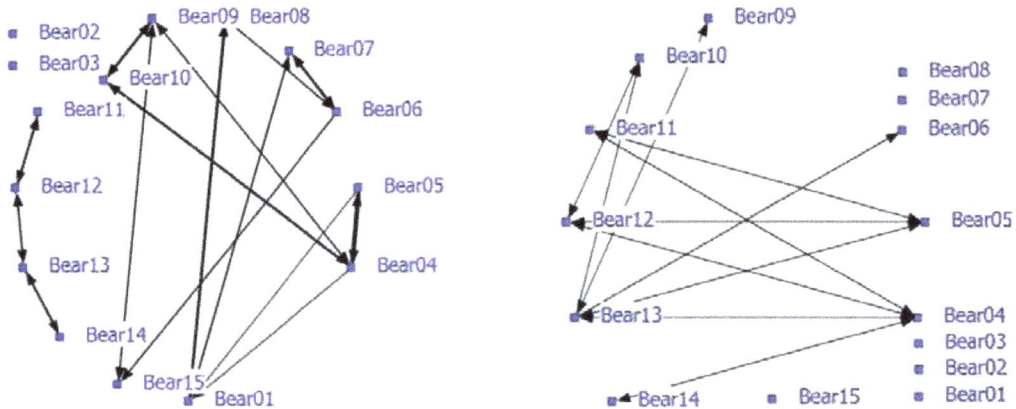

Bears 01 and 04 had the largest node degree and play a key role in the positive network (Table 5). Bears 02 and 03 have node degree zero, no betweenness and the highest farness score. The young bears (Bear11-14) are very distant from the other bears (Table 5: farness 169 and 171). Bears12 and 13 are cutpoints and important for the cohesion of the group of young bears. In nature, siblings often stay together after they have left their mother until they reach sexual maturity and become independent [54,55]. Bears 09 and 10 are associated; they knew each other before they came to the forest; both are blind and both like to play in the pond. Blind Bears 09 and 10 form a subgroup (Block 1) together with the very old male Bear01, Bears 04 and 05 (Block 2; betweenness high and farness low) and the females Bear06, Bear07 and Bear15.

Table 5. SNA characteristics showing individual and subgroup characteristics of brown bears in the LBE.

ID	Degree	Betweenness	Farness	Cutpoint	Block 1	Block 2	Block 3	Block 4	Block 5
Bear01	4	9.17	103	0	1	1	0	0	0
Bear02	0	0	210	0	0	0	0	0	0
Bear03	0	0	210	0	0	0	0	0	0
Bear04	4	8.33	103	0	1	1	0	0	0
Bear05	2	0	106	0	1	1	0	0	0
Bear06	3	4.17	106	0	1	0	0	0	0
Bear07	2	1.67	106	0	1	0	0	0	0
Bear08	2	1.67	106	0	0	1	0	0	0
Bear09	3	4.67	105	0	1	0	0	0	0
Bear10	2	0	107	0	1	0	0	0	0
Bear11	1	0	171	0	0	0	0	0	1
Bear12	2	2	169	1	0	0	0	1	1
Bear13	2	2	169	1	0	0	1	1	0
Bear14	1	0	171	0	0	0	1	0	0
Bear15	2	3.33	106	0	1	0	0	0	0
Average	2.00	2.47	136.53	0.13	0.53	0.27	0.13	0.13	0.13

For cutpoint and blocks: 0 = no and 1 = yes

The stability of the social network is shown by the positive significant correlations between the unlimited NN-matrices (N = 3491) on subsequent days and between relations on Days 1 and 10 (Table 6). Furthermore, the correlation between NN-matrices based on a maximum NND of 5 meters (N = 637) is also strongly positive (Table 6).

Table 6. Matrix correlations between NN-matrices based on daily nearest neighbor observations in brown bears for a period of 10 days. The last column shows the correlation between the first (1) and last day (10).

Days	1~2	2~3	3~4	4~5	5~6	6~7	7~8	8~9	9~10	1~10
Pearson's r	0.77	0.79	0.78	0.82	0.75	0.70	0.83	0.73	0.75	0.69
P-value	<0.001	<0.001	<0.001	<0.001	<0.001	<0.001	<0.001	<0.001	<0.001	<0.001
NND ≤ 5m	0.78	0.77	0.53	0.84	0.74	0.62	0.85	0.70	0.69	0.75
P-value	<0.001	<0.001	<0.001	<0.001	<0.001	<0.001	<0.001	<0.001	<0.001	<0.001

Both series of positive significant correlations show the stability of NN-locations or possible territories of the brown bears and the stability of positive associations or preferences between the brown bears (Table 6). Despite the fact that bears are generally considered solitary, they might have preferred places (territories) and individuals as nearest neighbors. This is in agreement with a simple social organization in brown bears as described in high-density gatherings during salmon-fishing [49].

4.3. Management

Although brown bears are in most cases solitary animals, some strong positive associations between bears are observed in this forest group, although the network densities are low. The unlimited NND network might be based on the locations, home ranges or territories the bears occupy in the bear forest that have a more fixed position than expected. The networks based on NND of a maximum 5 meters indicate that the individuals have positive and negative associations or preferences. This implies that management of removals of bears or cleaning the area has to be aware of the social and positional relations; the social structure of the bear group has also to be taken into consideration for feeding (at different locations) and cleaning of the enclosure. In traditional zoo enclosures bears are probably unable to establish home ranges or territories. LBEs have the advantage of providing more space for the bears, but the opportunity to establish a fixed home range or territories can imply a disadvantage. An adult strategy of allowing solitary territoriality and a juvenile strategy of social clustering with mobility may provide the best options to avoid fights and injuries. The available space might still be too limited, restricting the opportunity to roam around, avoid or even escape other bears. Brown bear welfare may be ameliorated when the density of bears is low and enough space per bear is available.

5. Example#3: Indoor Laying Hens—Video Observation of Nearest Neighbor

The social structure of the ancestors (red jungle fowl) of laying hens (*Gallus gallus domesticus*) is not precisely clear, but hens live in small groups that may be territorial [56]. They have strong preferences for specific habitats and are seen mostly (80%) alone or in some cases in very small groups [57]. Based on their behavior in the wild, the social network of laying hens might be a group of individuals with few relations or even solitary individuals when housed together. Recently, it was investigated whether or not hens establish friendships [21] or associate for other reasons [58,59]. No consistent evidence was forthcoming from these studies of hens actively preferring others in their choice of companions or resource area. Laying hens cluster considerably in all kinds of environments [59]. Broiler chickens were more socially attracted than aversive/avoidant [60], but stocking density will play a large role in social associations [61]. The question remains whether or not hens grouped together function as individuals indifferent to each other or whether they have closer friendships within the group. As domestication changed aspects of the behavior of the chicken such as contra-freeloading [62], aspects of the social behavior might also be changed. Description of the social network of laying hens in captivity may display a social network, mismatches with networks seen in the wild and provide solutions for damaging behavior such as feather pecking [13]. Two specific hypotheses were investigated: (1) the social network of laying hens shows relatively many unconnected and solitary individuals, and (2) the overall social network of laying hens is correlated with feather pecking in the focal hens.

5.1. Materials and Methods

In this study recordings were used from a study on facility demand or use of commodities in laying hens [63]. For this research, eight Bovans Goldline commercial hens aged between 23 and 28 weeks were used. The hens were identified with a 'backpack' labeled with different symbols. The laying hens were housed in a pen, with the dimensions of 2.97 × 4.60 meters, at the experimental farm of Schothorst Feed Research BV (Lelystad, the Netherlands). The pen consisted of a central grid and litter area and contained eight nesting boxes (with a single perch in front of the entrances) at one end, three perches at the other end and two round feeders and one round drinker in the middle. Food and water were always available. Five continuous 24-hr video recordings of the hens were used from November 2006, recorded from above with an analogue camera situated in the middle of the pen. There were 16 hours of light in the pen per day. Scans were made every 10 minutes. This provided 96 scans per day and 480 scans per hen in total. Each scan included the nearest neighbor (NN), the nearest facility and the behavior of the focal hen. Nearest neighbor distances were not measured. Hens that were not visible were noted as Not Seen (NS). The facilities were the nest perch (NPerch), drinking area (Drink), feeding area (Feed), grid area (Grid), litter area (Litter), nests (Nest) and perches (Perch). A NN-matrix (1-mode SNA) and a hen-nearest facility matrix (2-mode SNA) were calculated. Subsequent analysis of the NN-matrix was as described in Paragraph 2 (General Methods).

5.2. Results and Discussion

Relatively few significant nearest neighbors were found, so the density of the positive network was low at 0.16 (Figure 3; left graph). The graph shows some strong bonds especially between Hen5-Hen8, Hen1-Hen5 and Hen1-Hen7. The density of the negative network was lower (0.11). In the socio-negative graph, Hen1 displays the most connections often directed towards Hen8 (Figure 3; right graph). In socio-positive as well as in negative relationships, Hen1 may play a key role and may be important for the welfare in the group.

Figure 3. Social network of hens in an intensively managed indoor pen (positive network in left graph and negative network in right graph).

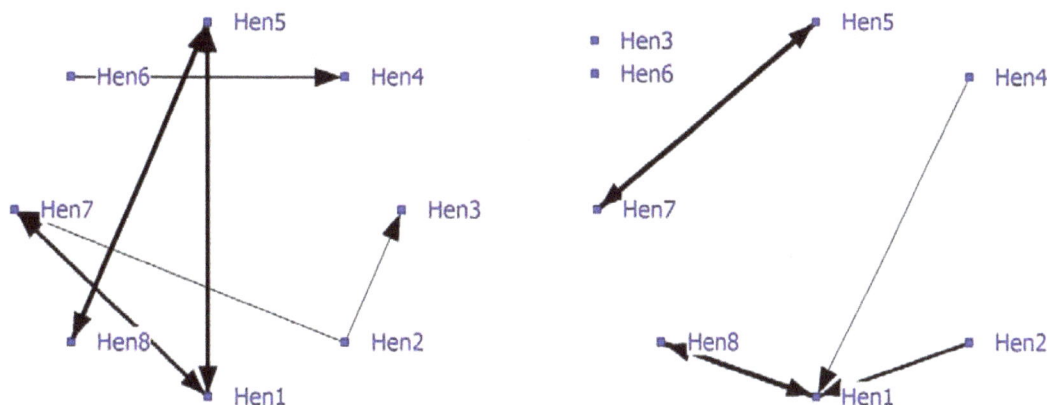

The importance of the individuals to the positive network is shown in individual and subgroup parameters (Table 7). Overall a low node degree was observed. Hen1 and Hen7 have the highest betweenness and the lowest farness within the network. Hen1 is also a cutpoint and connects Block3 (Hen1 and Hen7) with the hens in Block2 (Hen1 and Hen5). The other cutpoint is Hen5 who determines the relationship between Hen1 and Hen8. Subgroups based on cutpoints indicate three pairings of laying hens. Hens3, 4 and 6 are the most isolated hens in this group, having low degree, low betweenness, high farness and no subgroup participation.

Table 7. SNA characteristics showing individual and subgroup characteristics of laying hens in an indoor pen.

ID	Degree	Betweenness	Farness	Cutpoint	Block 1	Block 2	Block 3
Hen1	2	6	33	1	0	1	1
Hen2	2	4	35	0	0	0	0
Hen3	1	0	39	0	0	0	0
Hen4	1	0	57	0	0	0	0
Hen5	2	4	35	1	1	1	0
Hen6	1	0	57	0	0	0	0
Hen7	2	6	33	0	0	0	1
Hen8	1	0	39	0	1	0	0
Average	1.50	2.50	41.00	0.25	0.25	0.25	0.25

For cutpoint and blocks: 0 = no and 1 = yes

The NN-matrixes of subsequent days are significantly positively correlated and display the stability of the social network of the laying hens (Table 8).

Table 8. Matrix correlations between NN-matrices of subsequent days in laying hens for 5 days. The last column shows the correlation between the first (1) and the last day (5).

Days	1~2	2~3	3~4	4~5	1~5
Pearson's r	0.41	0.51	0.43	0.41	0.60
P-value	*0.009*	*0.002*	*0.005*	*0.014*	*0.000*

Laying hens show at least a number of stable individual associations, positive and negative. Whether they have friends [21] or not, or associate for other reasons [58,59] should be investigated further. The reason for this is that our study uses nearest neighbor analysis without a distance criterion and other studies have used the criterion that a hen is only a nearest neighbor when within a single bird-length of the focal hen [21]. Furthermore, in other research some specific periods of day and night were recorded while in the current study only daylight periods were recorded. The few significant associations found in captive conditions are in agreement with small groups of red jungle fowl associating under natural conditions [56,57]. Video recordings disclosed some limitations. The hens wore 'backpacks' with a symbol but often the hens flapped their wings and covered the symbol rendering them unrecognizable. With certain hens this happened quite often, affecting measurement reliability between hens. In future, this could be prevented by using an alternative recognition method. The hens were also less visible in the corners of the pen (this was probably due to the capability of the video or computer equipment).

In addition to the nearest neighbor information, the behavior of the focal hen was recorded. The focal hens feather pecked 93 times when scanned. Hen5 (23), Hen4 (18), Hen2 (15) and Hen7 (14) showed most feather pecking, while Hen2 (40) and Hen1 (28) were most often the nearest neighbor and probably victims of feather pecking. The NN-matrix while the actor was feather pecking (N = 93) was significantly correlated (R = 0.30, P = 0.027) with the total NN-matrix (N = 2584), indicating that the overall NN-matrix might be influenced by the feather pecking relations.

5.3. Management

The social structure of laying hens based on nearest neighbor data may be relevant for understanding and reducing problem behavior in (large) flocks of laying hens. Behavior was scanned at sampling moments but not continuously (*i.e.*, feather pecking FP). The associations found in the social positive and negative networks are not in agreement with the preliminary data. Hen1 displays no FP and is more often than expected the NN in the positive network of Hen5 who shows most FP. In the near future, feather pecking interactions should be measured and related with positive and/or negative networks based on NN-matrices in laying hens. Previous research with these laying hens attempted to determine their facility requirements using discrete-event modeling and facility capacity under different housing environments [63]. SNA can also include facility associations alongside individual associations. The positive 2-mode hen-facility network depicts a number of hens (Hen1, Hen2, and Hen8) that show no preference (as nearest neighbor) towards facilities (Figure 4; left graph). Hens6 and 7 are more often in the vicinity of food. The 2-mode negative hen-facility network indicates that these hens are found less frequently in the vicinity of the perch (Hen7) and litter (Hen6) (Figure 4; right graph). Significant association between animals and facilities may improve our understanding of 1-mode networks and probably be combined in future research and management.

Figure 4. Affiliation (2-mode) network of eight hens and five commodities based on significant positive associations (left graph) or significant negative associations (right graph).

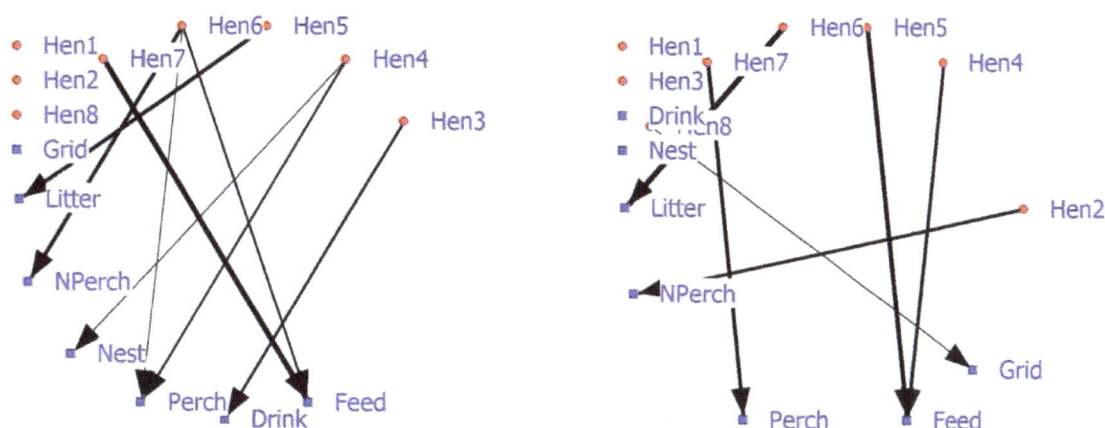

In conclusion, 2-mode hen-facility networks show associations that are relevant for poultry farmers and managers. Information about (changes in) the associations of individuals with other individuals, facilities or events (f.i. own behavior or that of others) in the environment can be visualized and provide support to improve management of captive animals. A combination of 1-mode and 2-mode social networks provides a potential tool to estimate and judge social and facility demands of laying hens [64,65].

6. Example#4: Indoor Veal Calves—Automated Recording of Location

Under natural conditions, during the first two weeks of life, calves (*Bos taurus*) develop a strong life-long bond with their dam through suckling, grooming and vocalization. Occasionally, a dam may leave her calf in a "crèche" of peers [66]. On commercial farms cow and calf are usually separated within three days after birth. Modern on-farm dairy management is focused on productivity performance based on high stocking densities, early weaning and hand-rearing. The innate urge of the calf for social interaction is neglected. Current housing systems restrict normal behavior and communication with conspecifics and may compromise calf welfare [67–69]. Social requirements and capabilities are especially relevant to the interpretation of veal calf welfare whether single housed, small group-housed (five–seven individuals) or in larger groups (40–80 individuals) [70]. Recently, it is has been shown that calves appear to form preferential relationships before they are 3.5 months old. Therefore, housing cattle together from an early age could be beneficial [71]. For management purposes, the following hypotheses were investigated: (1) veal calves form a social network under intensive housing conditions based on preferences of nearest neighbors, *i.e.*, a positive social network, (2) group-housed calves of 3.5 month show stable associations, and (3) automated measurement of calf locations facilitates fast and precise social network analysis.

6.1. Material and Methods

Our study was performed with 10 Holstein-Friesian calves (six males/four females) aged 3 to 4 months (bodyweight 88–138 kg) at the Dairy Campus experimental farm (Leeuwarden, The Netherlands). The calves were housed in a pen consisting of a lying area (20 m^2) with 12 cubicles, a walking area

(25 m^2) with a slatted floor and a feeding fence with 11 places. Individual location registration was performed per second from March 22 until April 17, 2013. This positioning determination system has been described previously [72]. Briefly, the system consists of receivers, transmitters and a processing computer, which together determine the position of each calf. The transmitters are placed at fixed locations throughout the barn, with a maximum distance of approximately 25 meters. The receivers are attached to the collar of the calves. The receiver determines the strength of the signal from each transmitter and sends this information to the processing unit. Signal loss is correlated with the distance between objects. These distances are used to calculate the position of the calves in the pen. Location is expressed as x- and y-coordinates in relation to the original location in the upper left corner of the barn where the pen is situated. Coordinate data became available per second and was corrected in a smoothing procedure [72]. Calf location was stored in the memory and adjusted when a subsequent position was recorded. Calculations were made of nearest neighbor and facility proximity every second. Data was sampled at a 10-minute interval to provide a NN-matrix based on observations of activity, feeding and lying [73]. Data were analyzed per day excluding the dark period (21–6 hrs.), when calf activity was low.

6.2. Results and Discussion

A complete social network analysis was performed involving all data not limited by NND (see Example #2 brown bears). The positive network has a density of 0.22 and the negative network a density of 0.23. Data showed that often only one calf was eating and the others were lying down. In that case the nearest neighbor was one of the lying calves depending on the eating position. The social network was recalculated using only NN-pairs with a NND of less than 1 meter. The unlimited NN-matrix (N = 17,330) correlated significantly positively (R = 0.95, P < 0.0001) with the NN-matrix using NN-pairs of NND < 1 meter (N = 11,429). The sociogram of both analyses is essentially the same; the sociogram of positive calf associations at less than 1 meter is shown within the group of ten calves (Figure 5; left graph). All calves displayed positive relationships, mostly two-way and sometimes one-way (Calf0-Calf3 and Calf2-Calf3). The positive and negative network densities are 0.23. The same amount of significant negative associations was found between the calves (Figure 5; right graph).

Figure 5. Social network of veal calves (NND < 1 meter) in an indoor intensively managed group (left: positive network, right: negative network).

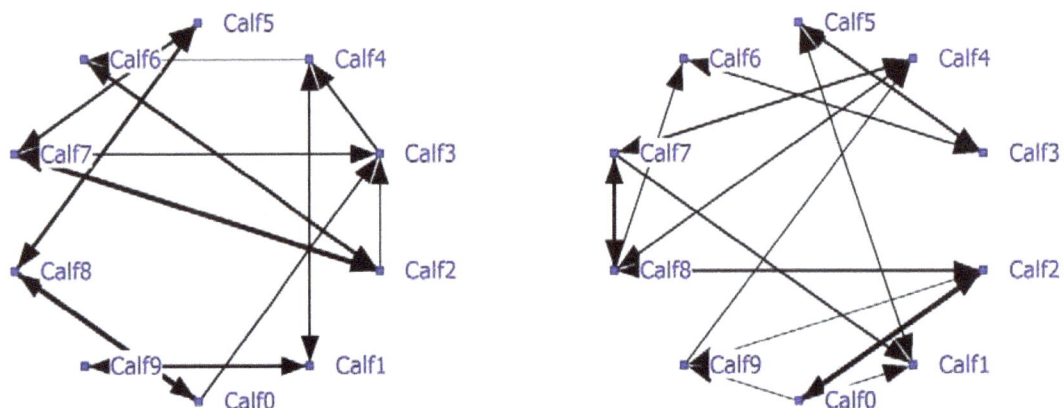

Calf03 has the highest node degree and thus most connections with other calves and is important to the group social structure (Table 9). Its betweenness is the highest and its farness the lowest of the group. Calf03 is a member of subgroup Block1 including eight of the 10 calves. Calf01 and Calf04 are cutpoints and thus essential connectors for the three subgroups found, especially with regard to the somewhat isolated Calf09. If the cutpoints are removed, the social network falls apart and Calf09 becomes totally isolated.

Table 9. SNA characteristics showing individual and subgroup characteristics of veal calves in an indoor stable.

ID	Degree	Betweenness	Farness	Cutpoint	Block 1	Block 2	Block 3
Calf0	2	5.167	30	0	1	0	0
Calf1	2	8	33	1	0	1	1
Calf2	3	3.667	29	0	1	0	0
Calf3	4	17.667	25	0	1	0	0
Calf4	3	15.333	27	1	1	1	0
Calf5	2	1.833	33	0	1	0	0
Calf6	2	1.5	31	0	1	0	0
Calf7	3	6.833	28	0	1	0	0
Calf8	2	1	35	0	1	0	0
Calf9	1	0	41	0	0	0	1
Average	2.40	6.10	31.20	0.20	0.80	0.20	0.20

For cutpoint and blocks: 0 = no and 1 = yes

Group stability is indicated by the correlations of NN-matrices between sample days (Table 10). Only Days 5 and 6 correlate significantly for the social network based on all data. The network structure appears to differ almost daily. Despite the indication of significant nearest neighbors, the overall analysis displays that the calves seem to have no preferred conspecifics. The observed network may be biased and based only on durations of cubicle lying behavior during long periods when the nearest neighbor is the same individual. In that case, calf location is relevant to the social structure. When the data are limited for only NND of 1 meter or less, the correlation between days remains generally not significant (Table 10). Only the correlation of the NN-matrices of Day 4 and Day 5 is significant, but negative. The almost complete lack of correlations between days places serious doubt on the existence of stable social relations within the group.

Table 10. Matrix correlations between matrices based on daily nearest neighbor observations of veal calves for 12 days. The last column shows the correlation between the first and the last day.

Days	1~2	2~3	3~4	4~5	5~6	6~7	7~8	8~9	9~10	10~11	11~12	1~12
Pearson's r	-0.09	0.00	0.15	-0.15	0.31	0.05	0.02	0.15	0.13	0.06	0.13	0.04
P-value	0.700	0.496	0.167	0.840	*0.024*	0.358	0.435	0.154	0.175	0.320	0.187	0.396
NND ≤ 1 m	-0.01	0.01	0.18	-0.32	0.20	0.07	0.04	0.14	0.09	0.07	0.15	−0.05
P-value	0.487	0.457	0.136	*0.011*	0.099	0.304	0.37	0.178	0.287	0.31	0.158	0.591

The claim that calves are capable of forming relationships within 3.5 months of age is challenged by the above findings [71]. Summarized over 12 days, the calves seem to have preferred neighbors, but the low non-significant day-to-day correlations show that these preferences are weak or non-existent.

6.3. Management

A positive and negative network was observed, but the day-to-day correlations were low and mostly not significant. This finding indicates that the stability of the social network is low or even that the networks may be based on chance caused by associations between calves using the same cubicles on consecutive days. In which case, location becomes very relevant for the interpretation of nearest neighbors in the same way as was found in the brown bear network, where fixed locations or territorial behavior were important factors. Especially for group-housed veal calves, natural management and consequent improvement of calf welfare, research in the day-to-day social network of the calves is crucial, and housing must be changed to facilitate social behavior and preferred associations between the calves.

In addition, facility usage is an important factor in on-farm management, as seen earlier in the laying hen example. The 2-mode SNA for veal calves indicates that in the positive network, half of the calves do not associate with a facility, while three calves display, above expectation, association with the slatted floor and two calves association with the cubicles (Figure 6; left graph). The negative calf-facility network indicates that three of the five calves (Calf8, Calf9 and Calf0) do not associate in a negative way with the facilities (Figure 6; right graph). Calf6 and Calf7 are found less frequently than expected in the cubicles and Calves1, 2 and 3 occupy the slatted floor less frequently than anticipated.

Figure 6. Social network of veal calves in an indoor intensively managed group (left: positive network, right: negative network).

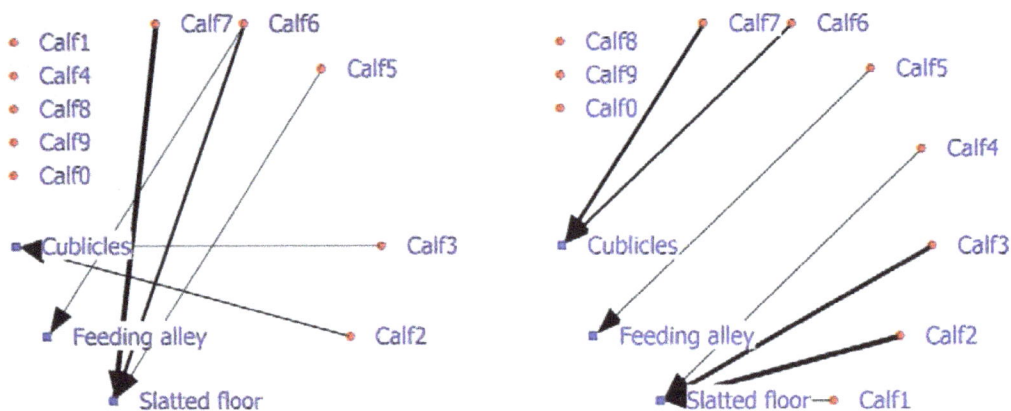

7. General Discussion

We used significant associations and dissociations based on standardized residuals of nearest neighbor frequencies as input for weighted positive or negative Social Network Analysis. This combination of old and modern methods is in our opinion suitable for the quick analysis of welfare-related problems. Replications of this method and comparison with different association measures or indices are needed to evaluate the method.

Information concerning nearest neighbors allows determination of significant associations between animals and between individuals and their environment. From our analysis, it is clear that this information remains insufficient. Validation is essential to the interpretation of the network, as is the location of each individual. We employed classic methods such as MatMan™ to find more individual and welfare related parameters. Most SNAs were performed with large datasets and based on un-weighted (1-0) edges between nodes. For small groups with small datasets, weighted SNA is probably more powerful. UciNet has some, albeit limited, power to analyze such weighted networks. Additional software for analyzing weighted social networks has only recently become available and is still under development [74,75]. Visualizing the observed network with NetDraw using weighted links or edges (SR) is helpful to judge the social network of small groups and can be used in management applications. The above examples show that SNA and knowledge concerning the social network of animals are relevant to the management and welfare of captive animals.

Removal of animals from groups provides knowledge of the animals' urges for social relationships and needs of the removed animal. The needs of the remaining animals must also be taken into consideration, for instance when an animal is removed, it may be crucial to the social structure or even create a cutpoint (breaking point) in the structure. Similar reasoning applies to introduction of animals into groups. We provide examples of networks based on nearest neighbor information. In horses, we found some indication that the positive network was indeed an important stimulant for individual welfare [48]. In the other examples no validation was observed. Fixed positions of animals in the enclosure or territorial behavior hamper the interpretation of the positive network in relation to welfare (e.g., bears and possibly the calf example). In order to reduce the influence of location preferences and fixed positions, the bear network was recalculated using a maximum NND of 5 meters and the calf network was recalculated using a maximum NND of 1 meter. These recalculated networks did not differ greatly from the complete networks using NN and unlimited NNDs. This also applies to negative networks and to the interpretation of negative effects on animal welfare. In calves, no day-to-day correlations between nearest neighbor matrices were observed, so consequently the resulting SNAs were difficult or impossible to interpret. It is possible that there is a social structure that is unstable or only stable for very short periods. Comparison between these findings and information from nature and literature is crucial to the welfare management of captive animals (see calves and crèches). At present, comparison of all the different housing and management conditions is impossible but may be possible in future, as more data from more species and more housing conditions become available. Automated measurement will be very helpful to facilitate applied Social Network Analysis. For the time being, the networks from the four examples have been compared using the densities of the positive and the negative networks provided (Table 11).

The socio-positive networks show densities between 0.12 and 0.23 and might be indicative of social (horse 0.21 and calf 0.23) or solitary (bear 0.12 and hens 0.16) species. The negative networks also show higher densities in the social species (horse 0.31 and calf 0.23) than the solitary species (bear 0.10 and hens 0.11). These findings are in line with the formulated hypothesis. Probably, when enough space is available, animals use the space to avoid non-preferred individuals. The total densities of both the positive and negative networks show that in social species approximately half of the associations between individuals are clearly positive or negative and half is not explicit (Table 11). That is lower in laying hens and much lower in brown bears where three-quarters of the associations between animals do not differ from a random distribution. The parameter %Positive allows an investigation of the relative positive density. The most positive social network was identified in laying hens, followed by bears (NND < 5 m), calves and the horse network. Individual brown bears avoid each other more according to the unlimited bear network. As stated earlier this may be caused by the fixed locations, home range or territories of the bears.

Table 11. Densities of the socio-positive and socio-negative networks of the four species, the total densities, the percentage of socio-positive of the total densities and the average correlation of the NN-matrices during trial periods.

Associations	Positive	Negative	Total	%Positive	Stability
Horse	0.21	0.31	0.51	40.53	0.54
Bear	0.16	0.37	0.53	30.63	0.77
Bear (NND < 5 m)	0.12	0.10	0.22	56.62	0.73
Chicken	0.16	0.11	0.27	60.01	0.44
Calf	0.22	0.23	0.46	48.78	0.07
Calf (NND < 1 m)	0.23	0.23	0.47	50.00	0.05

The stability of the SNs is shown in the average correlation between nearest neighbor matrices between days. Stability is highest in bears, followed by horses, laying hens and calves, where no stable social network was found.

However, there is room for improvement. Nearest neighbor identification is not always based on sufficient information for an adequate interpretation of the network data. Position, stability of the position and nearest neighbor distance is sometimes necessary for a correct interpretation of the SNs. In the first example, the nodes were labeled as mare or foal. In future, such node attributes may enhance the power of the SNA when information about, age, sex, weights or even personality is included as part of the SNA. This will become more likely with larger networks than the ones presented here. SNA provides opportunities to analyze the functioning of individuals in social groups in terms of approach and avoidance motivation and behavior. Using the SNA approach and avoidance tendencies in animals will provide additional information enabling determination of individual and group animal welfare.

8. Future Animal Management

Application of new technology, enabling simultaneous and more or less continuous localization of all individuals within a group, will make it possible to perform daily SNA. The parameters determined can then be translated into housing and management advice. In this context, parameters that reflect negative associations between individual animals or between individuals and their environment (facilities) become relevant, indicating that regrouping or removal of certain individuals can help animal welfare management. Social enrichment is one way of increasing welfare of solitary animals [76,77]. Social enrichment may strengthen a social network and increase individual welfare by introducing young animals [78]. Social enrichment by adding adults to social groups of juvenile animals may stabilize social networks of captives and increase welfare. In a situation where the social network is more or less stable from day to day, it can be determined how many and which animals have problems with the use of certain facilities such as places to rest, places to feed and other facilities within their environment. This information can lead to recommendations for adjusting the housing, available equipment and facilities. In addition, adjustments in the day-to-day management of the animals can be proposed, such as the feeding regime, or feed composition and quantity, and frequency of distribution. Current dairy farming practices already employ many different sensors to detect animals requiring special attention [79]. On-farm analyses of activity data are used to identify deviating activity, e.g., increased activity points to animals in estrus and reduced activity indicating health problems, such as locomotion. Daily information about the social network also allows following individual animals in time and thus providing an early warning of slow or sudden changes particularly in negative associations. It is interesting to consider whether or not the social network information can improve alerts for cows in estrus or with health problems. Application of location sensors in the management of farm animals is developing fast. These developments take place first in commercially important situations with large animals in small groups. In the near future, it is considered that it will become acceptable practice to apply sensors to pigs, and laying hens, if the analysis can be validated and the potential for animal welfare spin-off is made more apparent. Use of GPS or other location networks, will make SNA available for outdoor welfare management or even for feral animals. Certainly, intensive husbandry social network analysis has the potential to take on an important role in future animal management and welfare.

Acknowledgments

The authors wish to thank Andries Siepel and Lies Zandberg (Dartmoor ponies, Droevendaal, Wageningen), volunteers, José Kok and Corrian Rutte (brown bears, Bear forest, Rhenen), Erwin Mollenhorst, Nanda Ursinus and Diane de Snoo (laying hens, Schothorst), and N.V. Nederlandsche Apparatenfabriek, "Nedap", the Netherlands, for providing and installing the positioning system for calves, which was partly supported by the Dutch research program Smart Dairy Farming (www.smartdairyfarming.nl). The authors also thank the two anonymous reviewers for their valuable comments. A special thank you goes to Vincent Hindle for his help with the language revision.

Author Contributions

P. Koene designed, supervised, analyzed the experiments and drafted the manuscript. B. Ipema provided the veal calf information and contributed to writing the manuscript.

Conflicts of Interest

The authors declare no conflict of interest.

References

1. Hale, E.B. Domestication and the evolution of behaviour. In *The Behaviour of Domestic Animals*; Hafez, E.S.E., Ed.; Bailliére, Tindall & Cox: London, UK, 1962; pp. 21–53.
2. Koene, P. Behavioral ecology of captive species: Using behavioral adaptations to assess and enhance welfare of nonhuman zoo animals. *J. Appl. Anim. Welf. Sci.* **2013**, *16*, 360–380.

3. Krause, J.; Lusseau, D.; James, R. Animal social networks: An introduction. *Behav. Ecol. Sociobiol.* **2009**, *63*, 967–973.

4. Wey, T.; Blumstein, D.T.; Shen, W.; Jordan, F. Social network analysis of animal behaviour: A promising tool for the study of sociality. *Anim. Behav.* **2008**, *75*, 333–344.

5. Coleing, A. The application of social network theory to animal behaviour. *Biosci. Horizons* **2009**, *2*, 32–43.

6. Blonder, B.; Wey, T.W.; Dornhaus, A.; James, R.; Sih, A. Temporal dynamics and network analysis. *Methods Ecol. Evol* **2012**, *3*, 958–972.

7. Croft, D.P.; James, R.; Krause, J. *Exploring Animal Social Networks*; Princeton University Press: Princeton, NJ, USA, 2008.

8. Krause, J.; James, R.; Croft, D.P. Personality in the context of social networks. *Philos. T. R. Soc. B* **2010**, *365*, 4099–4106.

9. Krause, J.; Krause, S.; Arlinghaus, R.; Psorakis, I.; Roberts, S.; Rutz, C. Reality mining of animal social systems. *Trends Ecol. Evol.* **2013**, *28*, 541–551.

10. Krause, J.; Wilson, A.D.M.; Croft, D.P. New technology facilitates the study of social networks. *Trends Ecol. Evol.* **2011**, *26*, 5–6.

11. Haddadi, H.; King, A.J.; Wills, A.P.; Fay, D.; Lowe, J.; Morton, A.J.; Hailes, S.; Wilson, A.M. Determining association networks in social animals: Choosing spatial-temporal criteria and sampling rates. *Behav. Ecol. Sociobiol.* **2011**, *65*, 1659–1668.

12. Makagon, M.M.; McCowan, B.; Mench, J.A. How can social network analysis contribute to social behavior research in applied ethology? *Appl. Anim. Behav. Sci.* **2012**, *138*, 152–161.

13. Asher, L.; Collins, L.M.; Ortiz-Pelaez, A.; Drewe, J.A.; Nicol, C.J.; Pfeiffer, D.U. Recent advances in the analysis of behavioural organization and interpretation as indicators of animal welfare. *J. R. Soc. Interface* **2009**, *6*, 1103–1119.

14. Jones, H.A.C.; Hansen, L.A.; Noble, C.; Damsgard, B.; Broom, D.M.; Pearce, G.P. Social network analysis of behavioural interactions influencing fin damage development in atlantic salmon (salmo salar) during feed-restriction. *Appl. Anim. Behav. Sci.* **2010**, *127*, 139–151.

15. McCowan, B.; Anderson, K.; Heagarty, A.; Cameron, A. Utility of social network analysis for primate behavioral management and well-being. *Appl. Anim. Behav. Sci.* **2008**, *109*, 396–405.

16. Flack, J.C.; Girvan, M.; de Waal, F.B.M.; Krakauer, D.C. Policing stabilizes construction of social niches in primates. *Nature* **2006**, *439*, 426–429.

17. Carter, K.D.; Brand, R.; Carter, J.K.; Shorrocks, B.; Goldizen, A.W. Social networks, long-term associations and age-related sociability of wild giraffes. *Anim. Behav.* **2013**, *86*, 901–910.

18. Carter, K.D.; Seddon, J.M.; Frere, C.H.; Carter, J.K.; Goldizen, A.W. Fission-fusion dynamics in wild giraffes may be driven by kinship, spatial overlap and individual social preferences. *Anim. Behav.* **2013**, *85*, 385–394.

19. McComb, K.; Moss, C.; Durant, S. Elephant hunting and conservation—Response. *Science* **2001**, *293*, 2203–2204.

20. Williams, R.; Lusseau, D. A killer whale social network is vulnerable to targeted removals. *Biol. Lett.* **2006**, *2*, 497–500.

21. Abeyesinghe, S.M.; Drewe, J.A.; Asher, L.; Wathes, C.M.; Collins, L.M. Do hens have friends? *Appl. Anim. Behav. Sci.* **2013**, *143*, 61–66.

22. Boissy, A. Ethological research applied to farm animals: Reconciling animal welfare and production. *B Acad. Vet. France* **2012**, *165*, 137–148.

23. Boissy, A.; Manteuffel, G.; Jensen, M.B.; Moe, R.O.; Spruijt, B.; Keeling, L.J.; Winckler, C.; Forkman, B.; Dimitrov, I.; Langbein, J.; *et al.* Assessment of positive emotions in animals to improve their welfare. *Physiol. Behav.* **2007**, *92*, 375–397.

24. Rault, J.L. Friends with benefits: Social support and its relevance for farm animal welfare. *Appl. Anim. Behav. Sci.* **2012**, *136*, 1–14.

25. Morgan, K.N.; Tromborg, C.T. Sources of stress in captivity. *Appl. Anim. Behav. Sci.* **2007**, *102*, 262–302.

26. Murphy, M. Final discussion and conclusions. In *Social Stress in Domestic Animals*; Springer: Dordrecht, The Netherlands, 1990; Volume 53, pp. 295–307.

27. Rault, J.L.; Boissy, A.; Boivin, X. Separation distress in artificially-reared lambs depends on human presence and the number of conspecifics. *Appl. Anim. Behav. Sci.* **2011**, *132*, 42–50.

28. Koene, P. Feeding and welfare in domestic animals: A darwinistic framework. In *Feeding in Domestic Vertebrates, from Structure to Behaviour*; Bels, V., Ed.; CABI Publishing: Wallingford, UK, 2006; pp. 84–108.

29. Mollema, L.; Koene, P.; de Jong, M.C.M. Quantification of the contact structure in a feral cattle population and its hypothetical effect on the transmission of bovine herpesvirus 1. *Prev. Vet. Med.* **2006**, *77*, 161–179.

30. Koene, P. *Approach-Avoidance Conflict and Speed of Conflict Resolution*; Radboud: Nijmegen, The Netherlands, 1988.

31. Koene, P.; Vossen, J.M.H. A catastrophe model of approach-avoidance conflict. In *Viability of Mathematical Models in the Social and Behavioral Sciences*; Croon, M.A.; Van de Vijver, F.J.R., Eds.; Swets Zeitlinger: Lisse, The Netherlands, 1994; pp. 31–53.

32. Koene, P.; Vossen, J.M.H. Strain differences in rats with respect to speed of conflict-resolution. *Behav. Genet.* **1991**, *21*, 21–33.

33. Devries, H.; Netto, W.J.; Hanegraaf, P.L.H. Matman—A program for the analysis of sociometric matrices and behavioral transition matrices. *Behaviour* **1993**, *125*, 157–175.

34. Borgatti, S.P.; Everett, M.G.; Freeman, L.C. *Ucinet for Windows: Software for Social Network Analysis*; Analytic Tehnologies: Harvard, MA, USA, 2002.

35. Borgatti, S.P. *Netdraw Network Visualization*; Analytic Tehnologies: Harvard, MA, USA, 2002.

36. Hanneman, R.A.A.; Riddle, M. Introduction to social network methods. 2005. Available online: http://faculty.ucr.edu/~hanneman/nettext/ (accessed on 10 March 2014).

37. Cairns, S.J.; Schwager, S.J. A comparison of association indices. *Anim. Behav.* **1987**, *35*, 1454–1469.

38. Fagen, R.M.; Mankovich, N.J. 2-act transitions, partitioned contingency-tables, and the significant cells problem. *Anim. Behav.* **1980**, *28*, 1017–1023.

39. Koschutzki, D.; Lehmann, K.A.; Peeters, L.; Richter, S.; Tenfelde-Podehl, D.; Zlotowski, O. Centrality indices. *Netw. Anal.Methodol. Found.* **2005**, *3418*, 16–61.

40. Koschutzki, D.; Lehmann, K.A.; Tenfelde-Podehl, D.; Zlotowski, O. Advanced centrality concepts. *Netw. Anal. Methodol. Found.* **2005**, *3418*, 83–111.

41. Feh, C. Relationships and communication in socially natural horse herds. In *The Domestic Horse: The Origins, Development and Management of Its Behaviour*; Cambridge University Press: Cambridge, UK, 2005; pp. 83–93.

42. van Dierendonck, M.C.; Sigurjonsdottir, H.; Colenbrander, B.; Thorhallsdottir, A.G. Differences in social behaviour between late pregnant, post-partum and barren mares in a herd of icelandic horses. *Appl. Anim. Behav. Sci.* **2004**, *89*, 283–297.

43. Sundaresan, S.R.; Fischhoff, I.R.; Dushoff, J.; Rubenstein, D.I. Network metrics reveal differences in social organization between two fission-fusion species, grevy's zebra and onager. *Oecologia* **2007**, *151*, 140–149.

44. Lemasson, A.; Boutin, A.; Boivin, S.; Blois-Heulin, C.; Hausberger, M. Horse (equus caballus) whinnies: A source of social information. *Anim. Cogn.* **2009**, *12*, 693–704.

45. Tummers, B. Datathief III. 2006. Available online: http://datathief.org/ (accessed on 10 March 2014).

46. Perry, G.L.W. Sppack: Spatial point pattern analysis in excel using visual basic for applications (VBA). *Environ. Modell. Softw.* **2004**, *19*, 559–569.

47. Koene, P.; Zandberg, E.C.A. Social network stability and removals in horses. **2014**, in preparation.

48. Feh, C.; Demazieres, J. Grooming at a preferred site reduces heart-rate in horses. *Anim. Behav.* **1993**, *46*, 1191–1194.

49. Egbert, A.L.; Stokes, A.W. The social behaviour of brown bears on an alaskan salmon stream. *Ursus* **1974**, *3*, 41–56.

50. Bryan, H.M.; Darimont, C.T.; Paquet, P.C.; Wynne-Edwards, K.E.; Smits, J.E.G. Stress and reproductive hormones in grizzly bears reflect nutritional benefits and social consequences of a salmon foraging niche. *PLoS One* **2013**, *8*, doi:10.1371/journal.pone.0080537.

51. Grandia, P.A.; Van Dijk, J.; Koene, P. Stimulating natural behavior in captive bears. *Ursus* **2001**, *12*, 199–202.

52. Koene, P.; Ardesch, J.; Ludriks, A.; Urff, E.; Wenzelides, L.; Wittenberg, V. Interspecific and intraspecific social interactions among brown bears and wolves in an enclosure. *Ursus* **2002**, *13*, 85–93.

53. Koene, P. Adaptation of blind brown bears to a new environment and its residents: Stereotypy and play as welfare indicators. *Ursus* **1998**, *10*, 379–386.

54. Swenson, J.E.; Haroldson, M.A. Observations of mixed-aged litters in brown bears. *Ursus* **2008**, *19*, 73–79.

55. Swenson, J.E.; Franzen, R.; Segerstrom, P.; Sandegren, F. On the age of self-sufficiency in scandinavian brown bears. *Acta Theriol.* **1998**, *43*, 213–218.

56. Collias, N.E.; Collias, E.C.; Hunsaker, D.; Minning, L. Locality fixation, mobility and social organization within an unconfined population of red junglefowl. *Anim. Behav.* **1966**, *14*, 550–559.

57. Javed, S.; Rahmani, A.R. Flocking and habitat use pattern of the red junglefowl gallus gallus in dudwa national park, india. *Trop. Ecol.* **2000**, *41*, 11–16.

58. Asher, L.; Collins, L.M.; Pfeiffer, D.U.; Nicol, C.J. Flocking for food or flockmates? *Appl. Anim. Behav. Sci.* **2013**, *147*, 94–103.

59. Collins, L.M.; Asher, L.; Pfeiffer, D.U.; Browne, W.J.; Nicol, C.J. Clustering and synchrony in laying hens: The effect of environmental resources on social dynamics. *Appl. Anim. Behav. Sci.* **2011**, *129*, 43–53.

60. Febrer, K.; Jones, T.A.; Donnelly, C.A.; Dawkins, M.S. Forced to crowd or choosing to cluster? Spatial distribution indicates social attraction in broiler chickens. *Anim. Behav.* **2006**, *72*, 1291–1300.

61. Bokkers, E.A.M.; de Boer, I.J.M.; Koene, P. Space needs of broilers. *Anim. Welf.* **2011**, *20*, 623–632.

62. Lindqvist, C.E.S.; Schutz, K.E.; Jensen, P. Red jungle fowl have more contrafreeloading than white leghorn layers: Effect of food deprivation and consequences for information gain. *Behaviour* **2002**, *139*, 1195–1209.

63. Mollenhorst, H.; Kettenis, D.L.; Koene, P.; Ursinus, W.W.; Metz, J.H.M. Behaviour-based simulation of facility demand of laying hens. *Biosyst. Eng.* **2008**, *100*, 581–590.

64. Everett, M.G.; Borgatti, S.P. The dual-projection approach for two-mode networks. *Soc. Netw.* **2013**, *35*, 204–210.

65. Borgatti, S.P.; Everett, M.G. Network analysis of 2-mode data. *Soc. Netw.* **1997**, *19*, 243–269.

66. Phillips, C. *Cattle Behaviour and Welfare*; John Wiley & Sons: Hoboken, NJ, USA, 2008.

67. Thomas, T.J.; Weary, D.M.; Appleby, M.C. Newborn and 5-week-old calves vocalize in response to milk deprivation. *Appl. Anim. Behav. Sci.* **2001**, *74*, 165–173.

68. Flower, F.C.; Weary, D.M. Effects of early separation on the dairy cow and calf: 2. Separation at 1 day and 2 weeks after birth. *Appl. Anim. Behav. Sci.* **2001**, *70*, 275–284.

69. Weary, D.M.; Chua, B. Effects of early separation on the dairy cow and calf 1. Separation at 6 h, 1 day and 4 days after birth. *Appl. Anim. Behav. Sci.* **2000**, *69*, 177–188.

70. Bokkers, E.A.M.; Koene, P. Activity, oral behaviour and slaughter data as welfare indicators in veal calves: A comparison of three housing systems. *Appl. Anim. Behav. Sci.* **2001**, *75*, 1–15.

71. Raussi, S.; Niskanen, S.; Siivonen, J.; Hanninen, L.; Hepola, H.; Jauhiainen, L.; Veissier, I. The formation of preferential relationships at early age in cattle. *Behav. Process.* **2010**, *84*, 726–731.

72. Ipema, A.H.; van de Ven, T.; Hogewerf, P.H. Validation and application of an indoor localization system for animals. In Proceedings of 6th European Conference on Precision Livestock Farming, Leuven, Belgium, 10–12 September 2013; pp. 135–144.

73. Neisen, G.; Wechsler, B.; Gygax, L. Choice of scan-sampling intervals-an example with quantifying neighbours in dairy cows. *Appl. Anim. Behav. Sci.* **2009**, *116*, 134–140.

74. Opsahl, T.; Panzarasa, P. Clustering in weighted networks. *Soc. Netw.* **2009**, *31*, 155–163.

75. Opsahl, T.; Agneessens, F.; Skvoretz, J. Node centrality in weighted networks: Generalizing degree and shortest paths. *Soc. Netw.* **2010**, *32*, 245–251.

76. Schepers, F.; Koene, P.; Beerda, B. Welfare assessment in pet rabbits. *Anim. Welf.* **2009**, *18*, 477–485.

77. Reinhardt, V.; Houser, W.D.; Eisele, S.G.; Champoux, M. Social enrichment of the environment with infants for singly caged adult rhesus-monkeys. *Zoo Biol.* **1987**, *6*, 365–371.

78. Stradi, I.; Spiezio, C.; Sala, L. Infants in a colony of captive chimpanzees: Social enrichment? *Folia Primatol.* **2011**, *82*, 281.

79. Rutten, C.J.; Velthuis, A.G.J.; Steeneveld, W.; Hogeveen, H. Invited review: Sensors to support health management on dairy farms. *J. Dairy Sci.* **2013**, *96*, 1928–1952.

4

Health and Welfare in Dutch Organic Laying Hens

Monique Bestman* and Jan-Paul Wagenaar

Louis Bolk Institute, Hoofdstraat 24, 3972 LA, Driebergen, The Netherlands;
E-Mail: j.wagenaar@louisbolk.nl

* Author to whom correspondence should be addressed; E-Mail: m.bestman@louisbolk.nl.

Simple Summary: Data on animal health and welfare and farm management during rearing and laying periods were collected from 49 flocks of organic laying hens in the Netherlands to establish how farms performed in terms of animal health and welfare and which factors affected health and welfare.

Abstract: From 2007–2008, data on animal health and welfare and farm management during rearing and laying periods were collected from 49 flocks of organic laying hens in the Netherlands. Our aim was to investigate how organic egg farms performed in terms of animal health and welfare and which farm factors affected this performance. The flocks in our study were kept on farms with 34 to 25,000 hens (average 9,300 hens). Seventy-one percent of the flocks consisted of 'silver hybrids': white hens that lay brown eggs. Fifty-five percent of the flocks were kept in floor-based housing and 45% of the flocks in aviaries. No relation was found between the amount of time spent outdoors during the laying period and mortality at 60 weeks. Flocks that used their outdoor run more intensively had better feather scores. In 40% of the flocks there was mortality caused by predators. The average feed intake was 129 g/day at 30 weeks and 133 g/day at 60 weeks of age. The average percentage of mislaid eggs decreased from three at 30 weeks to two at 60 weeks. The average mortality was 7.8% at 60 weeks. Twenty-five percent of the flocks were not treated for worms in their first 50 weeks. Flubenol[©] was applied to the flocks that were treated. Ten percent of the flocks followed Flubenol[©] instructions for use and were wormed five or more times. The other 65% percent were treated irregularly between one and four times. Sixty-eight percent of the flocks showed little or no feather damage, 24% showed moderate damage and 8% showed severe damage. The feather score was better if the hens used the free-range area more intensely, the laying percentage at 60 weeks was higher, and if they were allowed to go outside sooner after arrival on the laying farm. In 69% of the flocks, hens had peck wounds in the vent area: on average this was 18% of the hens. Keel bone deformations were found in all flocks, on average in 21% of the birds. In 78% of the flocks, an average of 13% of the hens had foot-sole wounds, mostly a small crust. Combs were darker in flocks that used the range area more intensively. More fearful flocks had lighter combs. We conclude that organic farms are potentially more animal friendly than other poultry systems based on the animal welfare benefits of the free range areas. However, we also observed mortality rates, internal parasites, keel bone deformities, and foot sole lesions on organic farms that were comparable to or worse than in other husbandry systems. It is unclear whether these 'remaining' problems can be attributed to housing or if they are the result of keeping high productive genotypes in an artificial environment. Organic farms use the same high productive genotypes as other husbandry systems.

Keywords: organic; free range; poultry health; poultry welfare; feather pecking; vent pecking; mortality; keel bone deformations; foot sole lesions; comb color

1. Introduction

The organic egg sector in the Netherlands increased from 150,000 hens on 40 farms in 2001 [1] to 2.1 million hens on 194 farms in 2011 [2]. The most important features of Dutch organic egg production are [3] a maximum group size of 3,000 birds, six birds per m^2 indoors, 4 m^2 per bird outdoors, 18 cm perch per bird, and one third of indoor floor surface covered with litter. Moreover, the hens are given organically grown feed. In 2008, this was 90% organic. In the Netherlands, there is an additional organic hen rearing regulation. Its most important features are a maximum stocking density of 24 birds per m^2 during the first seven weeks and ten birds per m^2 between 7–18 weeks of age, 7 cm perch per bird from seven weeks onwards, and access to free range starting from eight weeks. The main thing organic egg production has in common with free-range production is the free-range area. The main differences are the number of animals per m^2 (six in organic and nine in free-range), organic ingredients in the feed, and farm size (up to 18,000 in organic and up to 40,000 in free range).

Many characteristics of organic poultry husbandry apply to loose housing in general. In the near future, we expect that the number of egg production systems with loose housing will further increase. In Europe, traditional cages are already forbidden. In the United States, the two States of California and Michigan passed state laws to ban battery cages. Although some farmers who have to stop using battery cages will turn to enriched cages, many farmers will switch to loose housing systems. The resemblance of organic systems to other loose housing systems and the expected growth of the alternative egg market, make our results valuable for a larger group of stakeholders than the organic sector alone.

The most recent overview of how Dutch organic farms perform in terms of health and welfare is based on data from 2001 and 2002 [4]. The results of that study were obtained through manure samples and a questionnaire for farmers. No physical assessment of animals took place. The mean flock size was 1,840 (80–5,400), the mean mortality was 11.4% (0–21) and the main health problems were predators, piling, coli, endoparasites, infectious bronchitis, and brachyspira. In the United Kingdom, a 7% mean mortality was reported in 1997 as well as cannibalism and coccidiosis [5]. A German study in 1999 [6] that involved a physical assessment of slaughterhouse hens reported pododermatitis, keel bone deformations, endoparasites, and fatty livers. In 2001 a Swedish study [7] based upon a questionnaire for farmers with 12–1,700 hens found a 9% (1–60) mean mortality, cannibalism, endoparasites, red mites, and leg parasites as health problems. A 2001 study in Austria [8] found a 7.2% (0–32) mean mortality, endoparasites, infectious bronchitis, Salmonella and cannibalism as health problems in 500–700 bird flocks. A Danish study [9] of 18 flocks with 1,200–5,000 hens found a 22% (9–62) mean mortality that was mainly caused by Pasteurella, predatory attacks, and piling. Thirty-three percent of the Danish flocks had little or no feather damage and 22% had severe feather damage. Of course, the type of health problems reported depend on the research methods applied. Interviews with farmers reveal mortality, and physical assessment may reveal pododermatitis and keel bone deformities, whereas manure samples give information about endoparasites. Though this makes the studies mentioned difficult to compare, they do give an impression of the range of health and welfare issues for organic laying hens during a period when flock sizes were much smaller and there was no common European organic poultry keeping legislation.

Organic hen keeping has been subjected to many changes, both in terms of regulations and trends in poultry husbandry since the most recent publication in 2003 [4] about the health and welfare of Dutch organic laying hens. Since then, beak treatments have been banned, aviaries have been introduced next to ground stables, flock sizes and number of hens per farm have increased, percentages of organic ingredients in poultry feed have increased, a national regulation for organic hen rearing has entered into force, different hybrids and genotypes have been introduced, and farmers have started to pay more attention to an attractive and functional free-range area.

Furthermore, farmers with organic hens experienced higher mortality rates than those with barn systems and were keen to understand how the health and welfare of their animals could be optimized. They wanted to know which factors in the rearing period and laying period influenced animal health and welfare parameters. Research questions were: how are organic egg farms performing in terms of health and welfare? How are farm practices during rearing and laying related to hen health and welfare during the laying period?

2. Methodology

We sent an invitation to 128 farms that kept organic laying hens according to Skal standards. Skal is the Dutch organic certification body. All farms that expressed an interest were included in the study. Our aim was for 50 flocks to take part. This number was a compromise between costs and statistic demands. In order to achieve a minimum of 50 flocks, farms who did not respond to the initial invitation were actively approached by phone in alphabetical order using the Skal's address list. Once 50 flocks had joined the study, new flocks were no longer able to take part. The 25 rearing farms that were approached reared the 'study flocks'.

Different questionnaires were designed for egg farmers and rearing farmers. The questionnaires were based on questionnaires from earlier studies and were discussed with several experts: veterinarians, farmers, poultry researchers, the Dutch Animal Protection organization, poultry advisors, hatcheries, and the Ministry of Economic Affairs, Agriculture and Innovation. The questionnaires covered housing and management, hybrid type, flock size, number of birds per m^2, feed, feed intake, egg production, mortality, mislaid egg percentage, feather pecking damage, health problems, and use of the free-range area. Both open and multiple-choice questions were included. The egg farmer questionnaires were filled in by the researcher during farm visits which took place when the hens were between 50 and 60 weeks old. Rearing farmers received their questionnaires by letter post and filled them out themselves.

A bird assessment protocol for farm visits was developed based on the following criteria:

- scoring should be objective,
- scoring should not demand expensive laboratory work,
- scoring items should be characteristics that farmers can see or feel themselves. This ensured that the study and its results were easy to communicate with the study's target group, the farmers.

Table 1. Methods used for body condition scoring.

Indicator	Assessment method	Relevance to welfare
Comb color	Konica Minolta color reader CR-10; measures color and describes it using three parameters: L, A and B-value [1]. L-value ranges from 0 to 100. A-values range from -86 to + 98. B-value ranges from -108 to + 94 [2].	Several diseases and health problems can cause a paler comb. Farmers regard bright red combs as a sign of health.
Feather condition	1. Visual scoring identifying a featherless spot of at least 5 centimeters diameter on a hen's back (yes/no) 2. Visual scoring of flock pictures taken according to Tauson et al. [10]. Classification of scoring of 6 body parts on a scale from 1 (completely featherless) to 4 (no or few feathers missing) [3].	Featherless spots are caused by feather pecking. This is a sign of reduced welfare in both actor [11,12] and victim [13]. Feather pecking can be caused by several factors during the rearing and laying period.
Wounds	Visual scoring of wounds on back, vent and tail area (yes/no)	Skin wounds can be caused by pecking behavior or accidents. Wounds are a sign of reduced welfare and make a bird potentially more vulnerable to infections.
Abnormalities on foot soles	Visual scoring of foot soles by observer (normal/scab/abscess).	Foot soles can have wounds or infections, caused by abnormalities in housing and reduced resistance against diseases (see discussion).
Keel bone deformations	Palpation of keel bone: deformity yes/no. Deformities are defined as deviations from the normally straight line (lateral or dorso-ventral) or thickened sections.	Keel bone deformations can be caused by 'metabolic bone disease', accidents and resting on the keel during perches.
Body weight	Weighing scale in grams.	Body weight could be compared to breeding standards and uniformity within a flock could be calculated (see discussion).

[1] Available online: http://sensing.konicaminolta.asia/learning-center/meter-measurement/meter-spaces (accessed on 2 April 2014); [2] Available online: http://stackoverflow.com/questions/19099063/what-are-the-ranges-of-coordinates-in-cielab-meter-space (accessed on 2 April 2014); 3 For each flock one mean was calculated for all body parts from 50 scored hens. To make the Tauson scores more illustrative, three 'qualitative' categories were defined: no/little damage (Tauson score 3.1–4); moderate damage (Tauson score 2.1–3) and severe damage (Tauson score 1–2).

The birds were assessed between 50 and 60 weeks of age. Fifty birds were caught individually at each farm. In tame flocks, this was done by hand while walking through the flock and in shy flocks by cornering the birds using a 'catch crate'. The indicators listed in Table 1 were determined for each individual bird. To avoid inter-observer bias, bird assessments on all the farms were done by the same researcher.

A manure sample was obtained by collecting 20 fresh droppings indoors. These were mixed and sent to the GD Animal Health Service (Deventer, the Netherlands). The sample was analyzed using the McMaster flotation method for worm egg counts. Shell and yolk color measurements were done with a Konica Minolta color reader CR-10 on thirty first-grade eggs that were collected from each flock. Pictures were taken of flocks and housing. After individual birds were assessed, the fear level of the whole flock was assessed during the researcher's visit. This was done on a scale from one (calm) to 10 (showing fearful behavior by flying up several times). The one, five and 10 on this scale were described and the observer made a rough estimate of the rest of the scale. Farmers scored health problem occurrence by indicating whether or not the flock had encountered a prelisted health problem (YES) in the flock or not (NO).

To estimate free-range use, the parameter Free Range Use (FRU) was calculated:

FRU = number of weeks free range is available (popholes open) in the period of 17–50 weeks of age × the maximum percentage of hens seen outside simultaneously under most optimal conditions (estimated by the farmer)

Since the flocks were 50–60 weeks old when we enquired about maximum range use, the percentages covered three seasons and all hours of the day. This prevented a 'snapshot' impression of range use.

All data were entered into an Excel spreadsheet. Statistics were calculated using the General Linear Model procedure (regression analysis). The RSEARCH procedure to find meaningful models ('all subset regression') was our starting point. Because R^2 was relatively low in most of these models, we moved on to linear regression for single factor relationships. In the regression analysis, relations were considered as not meaningful if the adjusted R^2 was less than 20. The two-sample t-test (unpaired, two-sided) and correlations (the two-sided test of difference from zero) were also used. GenStat for Windows, 13th edition, VSN International Ltd. (2010) was used to calculate all statistics.

3. Results

Results were collected from 49 organic laying flocks on 43 farms. Some of these farms volunteered after receiving our invitation letter. The rest joined when the letter was followed by a phone call. We received information about the rearing period of 35 of these 49 flocks.

3.1. Number and Size of Farms

Five of the 49 flocks were kept on four farms with less than 500 hens. Forty-four flocks were kept on 39 farms with more than 500 hens. The average number of hens on all farms was 9,300 (min 34–max 25,450). Table 2 shows the distribution of the number of hens per farm.

Three egg farms had their own hen-rearing facilities.

Table 2. Distribution of farm sizes.

Size of farms	Number of farms	Percentage of farms
0–100	1	2
101–500	4	8
501–1,000	0	0
1,001–5,000	7	14
5,001–10,000	18	37
10,001–15,000	14	29
15,001–20,000	2	4
20,001–25,450	3	6
Total	49	100

3.2. Hybrids

The most-used hybrid was H&N Silver Nick (51%), followed by Hy-line Silver (20%), Hy-line Brown (10%) and Lohmann Brown Lite (8%). Most of the hens were so-called 'silvers': white- feathered hens that lay brown eggs.

3.3. Housing and Use of the Free Range Area

Twenty-two (45%) of the 49 flocks were kept in aviaries and 27 (55%) in a floor-based housing system (see Table 3). The latter had a grid floor with perches above a manure pit. Eleven of the 22 aviaries had a winter garden, of which 10 were 'regarded as stable area'. 'Regarded as stable area' means that the farmer includes its surface when calculating the number of hens allowed in the stable + winter garden combination. Such winter gardens do not provide additional space, but do provide 'different' space in terms of temperature and daylight. Twelve of the 27 floor-based stables had a winter garden, of which 11 were regarded as stable area.

Table 3. Distribution of housing systems.

Housing system	No of flocks	Winter garden yes/no
Aviary	22	11 yes 11 no
Floor	27	12 yes 15 no
Total	49	23 yes 26 no

Thirty-nine (80%) of the 49 flocks had less than 25% sheltered area in the form of bushes, maize or artificial structures in their outdoor ranging area. Seven flocks (14%) had 26–50% sheltered area, and three flocks (6%) had more than 50% sheltered area (see Table 4). 19 out of 48 flocks (40 %) had mortality by predators: 7 flocks by birds of prey (15%), 6 flocks by foxes (13%) and 6 flocks by both (13%).

Table 4. Amount of shelter in outdoor runs.

Percentage of surface covered with bushes, maize or artificial structures	Number of flocks	Percentage of flocks
<25	39	80
26-50	7	14
>50	3	6
Total	49	100

During the study, national avian influenza alerts resulted in five periods of decreed indoor confinement. Four of these periods were in autumn or winter and one of them was in the summer. Five of the 49 flocks were vaccinated against avian influenza. These flocks were allowed to range during the confinement periods. The hens that were allowed to range shortly after their arrival on the laying farm tended to range more between 50 and 60 weeks of age (correlation -0.33; $p = 0.03$). When hens were allowed to range, on average 62% of the birds in a flock were seen outside together.

Flocks that used the outdoor run more intensively, with higher FRU, had better feather scores (regression analysis; $R^2 = 25$; $p < 0.001$).

The more intensively hens used the outdoor run, the better farmers assessed their general health and performance (regression analysis; $R^2 = 18$; $p = 0.003$).

3.4. Technical Performance

Table 5 is an overview of production parameters at 30 and 60 weeks of age.

Table 5. Production parameters at 30 and 60 weeks of age.

Item	30 weeks Mean (min-max)	60 weeks Mean (min-max)
Feed intake (gram/hen/day)	129 (109–147)	133 (113–160)
Production (laying %)	91 (76–96)	80 (58–92)
Mislaid eggs (%)	3 (0–12)	2 (0–12)
Mortality (%)	2 (0–11)	7.8 (0–34)

Zero % mislaid eggs means 'close to zero'. Zero % mortality was found in one very small flock, where none of the hens died in their first 60 weeks. The one flock with 34% mortality was a 8,800-hen flock that got infected with the bacteria *Erysipelotrix*.

3.5. Body Weight

Calculations were done for the H&N Silver Nicks because this was the only genotype with enough available flocks. We found a relation between growth during the period of 7 to 11 weeks and body weight in the laying period at 50–60 weeks (regression analysis; $R^2 = 36$; $p = 0.005$): the faster the pullets grew during the middle of the rearing period, the higher their body weight was at a later age.

Table 6 shows mortality distribution.

Table 6. Distribution of mortality at 60 weeks of age.

Mortality	Number of flocks	Percentage
0–5	21	43
6–10	15	31
11–15	4	8
16–20	4	8
>20	1	2
Unknown	4	8
Total	49	100

Table 7 is a list of reported health problems. A health problem was defined as such if the farmer perceived it as a problem. Some problems were diagnosed by a veterinarian and some were not. Health problems were not quantified in terms of mortality or production loss.

Table 7. Presence of health problems.

Health problem	Number of flocks
E. Coli	18 (37%)
Red blood mites	16 (33%)
Infectious Bronchitis	15 (31%)
Piling	15 (31%)
Skin infections	11 (22%)
Multi systemic wasting syndrome	11 (22%)
Intestinal parasites	9 (18%)
Chronic gut infection (enteritis)	6 (12%)
Blackhead	5 (10%)
Fatty livers	2 (4%)
Botulism	1 (2%)
Amyloidosis	1 (2%)
Coccidiosis	0 (0%)

3.6. Intestinal Parasites in Relation to Anthelmintic Use

For one flock it was unclear whether it had been wormed. Therefore, results were available for 48 flocks. Twelve of 48 flocks (25%) were not wormed up to 50 weeks of age (see Table 8). Thirty-one flocks (65%) were wormed irregularly or less frequently than recommended with an anthelmintic producer (e.g., Flubenol$^{©}$ every 6 weeks). Only five flocks (10%) were wormed five or more times between 17 to 50 weeks of age. Table 8 shows egg count results. With regression analysis we did not find a meaningful relation between worming of a flock (yes/no) and % lay at 60 weeks (regression analysis; $R^2 = 15.2$; $p = 0.005$), or between worming of a flock (yes/no) and mortality at 60 weeks (regression analysis; $R^2 = 6.2$; $p = 0.731$).

Table 8. Number of anthelmintic treatments up until 50 weeks of age (n = 48).

	Number of flocks	Positive for Ascaridia and Heterakis	Positive for Capillaria	Positive for Coccidiosis	Positive for Syngamus
No treatment	12 (25%)	83%	25%	25%	0%
Irregular, less frequent than prescribed, *i.e.*, treated 1-4 times	31 (65%)	61%	19%	42%	0%
Treated 5 or more times	5 (10%)	0 (0%)	0%	3 (60%)	0%

3.7. Parasites and Egg Yolk Color

Yolk color measurements determined L-, A- and B-values. In a color series of slightly yellow to orange, the L-value decreases and both the A- and B-values increase. Flocks that were positive for Ascaridia or Heterakis had higher L-values, meaning a lighter yolk color ($p = 0.002$; two-sample t-test; 47 d.f.). Flocks that were positive for Capillaria also showed a higher L-value, which meant a lighter yolk color ($p = 0.035$; two-sample t-test; 47 d.f.).

3.8. Feather Pecking Damage

On average, 64% (minimum zero; maximum 100) of the hens in all 49 flocks had a featherless spot of at least five centimeters diameter on their backs. The score results using Tauson *et al.*'s [10] method of scoring six body parts of 50 hens are shown in Table 9. The scores between one and four were obtained following Tauson's protocol. In addition we defined qualitative categories to make the outcomes more illustrative. Tauson's scoring was done on the basis of photographs. Photographs that were of sufficient quality to score were available for only 37 flocks.

Table 9. Severity of feather damage according to Tauson *et al.* (2005).

Category	Number of flocks
No/little feather damage (Tauson score 3.1–4)	25 (68%)
Moderate feather damage (Tauson score 2.1–3)	9 (24%)
Severe feather damage (Tauson score 1–2)	3 (8%)
Total	37

Twenty-five of 37 flocks (68%) had little or no feather damage, nine flocks (24%) had moderate damage and three flocks (8%) had severe damage. The feather score was better (RSEARCH procedure (all possible subset selection; $R^2 = 52$) if the FRU was higher ($p = 0.003$), the laying percentage at 60 weeks was higher ($p = 0.007$), and the sooner the hens went outside after arrival on the laying farm ($p = 0.024$).

3.9. Vent Pecking

Peck wounds in the vent area were observed in 34 of 49 flocks (69%). On average, 18% (min two–max 50) of the birds in these 34 flocks had wounds in the vent area. It was not possible to make quantitative statements about wound severity as scores were based on wound presence (yes/no). Most of the wounds had an approximate diameter of 0.5 cm, a small amount was bigger (up to 2 cm diameter).

3.10. Keel Bone Deformations

Keel bone deformations were found in all 49 flocks. On average, 21% (min four–max 48) of the birds in a flock had a keel bone deformation: a lateral or dorso-ventral deviation, a thickened section or a combination. In our study farmers used either round metal or rectangular wooden perches. With regression analysis we did not find a relation between keel bone deformation and perch type (regression analysis; $R^2 = 11$; $p = 0.012$) or between keel bone deformation and aviary or floor-based housing (regression analysis; $R^2 = 11$; $p = 0.012$).

3.11. Foot Sole Lesions

Wounds on foot soles were observed in 38 of the 49 flocks (78%). On average, 13% (min two–max 48) of the birds in these flocks had such wounds. Since we scored hens on the basis of wound presence (yes/no), it is not possible to make quantitative statements on the severity of these wounds. The majority showed wounds of 0.2–0.5 cm diameter. Swellings that are characteristic for bumble foot were rarely observed. No relation was found between foot sole lesions and FRU (regression analysis; $R^2 = 11$; $p = 0.013$).

3.12. Comb Color

Comb color measurements entailed defining L-, A- and B-values. In a color series of pink to dark red, the L-value decreases and both A- and B-values increase. The hybrid type (with regression analysis) significantly explained the overall difference in comb color (L-value $R^2 = 29$, $p = 0.003$; A-value $R^2 = 24$; $p = 0.009$; B-value $R^2 = 46$, $p < 0.001$). Therefore, further calculations were only done for the most-used hybrid: H&N Silver Nick. A higher FRU was related to a lower L-value, thus darker combs (regression analysis; $R^2 = 29$; $p = 0.003$). Flocks that reacted more fearfully during our visits had higher L-values, thus lighter combs (regression analysis; $R^2 = 34$; $p = 0.003$). Flocks that tested positively for one or more intestinal parasites, tended to have a higher B-values, thus darker combs (t-test; $p = 0.036$).

3.13. Rearing

Data regarding the rearing period was available for 35 of the 49 flocks. Not all questionnaires on the rearing period were complete. Six of the 33 flocks (18%) were kept in cages during the first weeks of their lives. Three of those flocks were kept on 'pullet paper' without litter. Twenty-six (79%) of the 33 flocks had litter from day one. In loose housed rearing, the group size was 13,800 (n = 25 flocks). The average pullet density during the first four weeks was 21 pullets/m^2 (n = 33), with 8.5 as minimum and 33.5 as maximum. After four weeks, many flocks were given additional space, resulting in an average density of 14 pullets/m^2 (min 6.6 and max 27.5). For 33 flocks, there was data available regarding whether they had access to an outdoor run. Nine flocks had not been outside and 26 flocks had access to an outdoor run. The average age for first time access was 8.4 weeks. At 17 weeks, on average 28% of the animals from the 'outside flocks' was seen outside.

4. Discussion

The study incorporated data from 49 flocks on 43 farms. Some of the farms volunteered after receiving an invitation letter and the rest joined when the letter was followed by a phone call. It is possible that the farmers who volunteer to participate, are those who perform well. If this is the case, our results may overestimate the welfare situation on farms. Five of these 49 flocks were kept on four farms with less than 500 hens. Forty-four flocks were kept on 39 farms with more than 500 hens. According to Loefs [14] there were 107 farms with organic laying flocks in the Netherlands in 2008 and she only counted farms with more than 500 hens. Our 39 flocks represent slightly more than one third of the farms (39/107 = 36%).

4.1. Relation between Outdoor Run Use and Health and Welfare

We did not find any relation between the number of weeks that hens spent outside during the laying period and mortality at 60 weeks, nor was a relation found between the number of confinement periods and mortality at 60 weeks. However, several studies showed a higher mortality or a higher disease incidence in free-range or organic poultry compared to hens kept inside [15,16]. In 19 of 49 (39%) of our flocks there was mortality caused by predators. Other studies also reported mortality caused by predators. These studies focused on broilers [17] or they presented their results differently [18,19]. Therefore, it is not possible to compare these results to our results. However, all studies illustrate that losses caused by predators are a realistic risk of keeping free-ranging poultry. If mortality is a measure for bird welfare, then one could argue that hens on free-range farms have a reduced welfare. Flocks that used the outdoor run more intensively had better feather scores. If the amount of feather-pecking damage is used as a measure for hen welfare, then hens on farms where more hens use the free-range areas have a better welfare [20–23].

The more intensely hens used the outdoor run, the better the farmer assessed their general health and performance. Since we found this relation with regression analysis, there may not be a causal relation between the two parameters. Which health and performance aspects satisfy farmers regarding their hens remain unknown, but the relation shows that somehow good use of the outdoor run relates to good health and/or performance perceived by farmers.

4.2. Technical Performance

On average birds had a feed intake of 129 g/day (min 109–max 147) at 30 weeks and 133 g/day (min 113–max 160) at 60 weeks of age. The mean intake levels were within an acceptable range. The feed intake depends on ambient temperature, plumage condition, and housing system [24].

The mean number of mislaid eggs decreased during the laying cycle from three to two percent, which might be caused by adequate management interventions. The mean mortality of 7.8% at 60 weeks of age is difficult to compare with other studies, because these studies describe results of the entire laying cycle, which can be up to 70 weeks or more. Mortality is generally higher in alternative systems [25].

4.3. Body Weight

We found a relation between growth in the rearing period and body weight at 50–60 weeks: the faster the pullets grew during the middle of the rearing period (weeks of life 7–11), the higher was their body weight at later age. Although for several other aspects, a relation has been found between conditions in the rearing period and the laying period, for example feather pecking, we did not find literature specifically on laying hen body weight.

4.4. Intestinal Parasites in Relation to the Use of Anthelmintic

Depending on the number of anthelmintic treatments, a considerable number of flocks tested positively for internal parasites. We did not find a relation with production or mortality. For different reasons it is not clear whether zero tolerance of internal parasites is necessary. Firstly, a low infection level might not be harmful. Secondly, when a higher infection level is combined with other health problems, one could ask what came first: the other health problems, which made the birds vulnerable to parasites or the parasites that made the birds vulnerable to other health problems. In 1999, Thamsborg et al. [26] already found that the significance of infections in terms of disease and production losses on organic farms had not been assessed. Moreover, the GD Animal Health Service, a Dutch authority on farm animal health, has the following text on their website [27] 'not all internal parasite species are equally harmful' and 'treatment therefore is not always necessary'. They refer to 'your personal vet' for personal advice. Flubendazole is the only registered anthelmintic medicine against internal parasites in poultry, and parasites may become resistant to it. Therefore, zero tolerance in healthy flocks does not seem logical.

Flocks that were positive for Ascaridia or Heterakis had a lighter yolk color. Flocks that were positive for Capillaria also had a lighter yolk color. Although non-scientific on-line publications recognize this relation, we were unable to find scientific articles to support our findings. A general explanation seems to be that parasites damage the intestines, which in turn influences pigment intake.

4.5. Feather Pecking Damage

Sixty-four percent of the hens in all 49 flocks were found to have feather damage on their back when the first method was used. However, we found that 68% of the flocks had 'no or little' feather damage when Tauson's method was applied in combination with categories we defined to qualify the damage. The difference may be caused by the fact that a five-centimeter featherless spot on a hen's back qualifies as little damage if the rest of the hen's feathers are in good condition, which was mostly the case. As Tauson's method reflects variation better, we think that the method is more suitable than a quick scan of only one body part.

Twenty-five of 37 flocks (68%) showed no or little feather damage, nine flocks (24%) showed moderate damage and three flocks (8%) showed severe damage. The feather score was better if the free-range use was better, the laying percentage at 60 weeks was higher, and the sooner the hens went outside after arrival on the laying farm. A relation between better free-range use and better feather cover is also reported in other studies [20–23]. A free-range area can be considered as environmental enrichment. Other types of environmental enrichment, such as additional foraging materials [28], scattered grains [29], and elevated perches [30] are also associated with less feather pecking. Another explanation could be that if a flock is distributed over a larger area, the stocking density decreases. Lower stocking density (in combination with a smaller group size) is also associated with less feather pecking [31–33]. Concerning the relation between higher laying percentage and better feather cover, it is not clear if this is a causal relationship. There is not much literature to be found on this relation, although Hüber-Eicher and Sebö [34] found the same relation in Swiss commercial flocks.

4.6. Vent Pecking

In 34 of 49 flocks (69%) peck wounds were seen in the vent area. On average, 18% (min two–max 50) of the birds had wounds in the vent area. Most of them were about 0.5 cm in diameter, a small number of them was bigger, up to 2 cm. Pötzsch et al. [35] found that 36.9% of non-cage housed flocks in the UK were affected by vent pecking. However, this was based on the farmer's judgments obtained through voluntary questionnaires. Vent wounds are best observed by manually diagnosing individual hens. Lambton et al. [36], who did behavioral observations in 119 British flocks (barn, free-range and organic), observed vent pecking behavior in 24.8% of the flocks. According to Pötzsch et al. [35], vent pecking and feather pecking damage may be caused by shared common environmental risk factors.

4.7. Keel Bone Deformations

Keel bone deformations were seen in all 49 flocks. On average, 21% (min four–max 48) of the birds in a flock had a keel bone deformation: a lateral or dorso-ventral deviation, a thickened section or a combination. We are not sure how many of the deviations we observed were fractures, since we used the palpation method for our assessment instead of animal dissection. Wilkins et al. [37] compared palpation and dissection methods and concluded that in 91% of the cases palpation gave a correct result, assuming that the dissection method is the correct result. We are not sure whether the lateral and dorso-ventral deviations were the result of fractures or a slowly-developed curve. Wilkins et al. [37] found keel bone fractures in 36% to more than 80% of the animals in flocks kept in different housing systems. Gregory and Wilkins [38] found that 30% of 72-week old hens had a broken keel. Nicol et al. [39] found 52–59% of hens with keel breaks in commercial flocks in aviaries. In those studies, keel bone assessment was done on dissected hens. Compared to those studies, our 21% average of hens with a keelbone deviation (not all of them being a fracture) seems low. Twenty-one percent might be an underestimation of the real number of fractures.

In our study, farmers used either round metal or rectangular wooden perches. We did not find any relation between keel bone deformation and perch type. Nor was a relation found between keel bone deformation and aviary or floor-based housing systems.

4.8. Foot Sole Lesions

In 38 of 49 flocks (78%) wounds on foot soles were seen. On average, 13% (min two–max 48) of the birds in these flocks had foot sole wounds. The majority of them were 0.2–0.5 cm in diameter. Swellings characteristic of bumble foot were rarely observed.

Nicol *et al.* [39] measured foot damage in laying hens. They used a five-point scoring system with one meaning 'no lesions' and five meaning 'very poor foot condition with inflamed and/or bleeding lesions visible over much of the area'. The foot damage in their study never exceeded an average value of 1.5, thus staying between 'no lesion' and 'lesions which are clearly visible but of minor importance and/or frequency'. Although different assessment methods were applied, which means their results are difficult to compare with our results, we assume the results are about the same.

Tauson and Abrahamsson [40] showed that perch design was an important factor for bumble foot in laying hens. Hens in cages without perches had the best scores: no bumble foot at all. When hens from cages with four different perch designs were compared, those with the narrow perches had the best bumble foot scores and those with broader perches the worst. The narrow perches were narrow rectangular (35 mm wide) or flat/round (38 mm wide). The broader perches were plastic 'mushroom' (48 mm wide) and wooden wide rectangular (53 mm wide). The authors' explanation is that a good anatomical grip is not possible on broader perches and this results in too much pressure on the hen's foot at rest. Lay *et al.* [25] concluded that wet litter conditions and high ammonia litter content in litter could cause footpad dermatitis in hens, which could be followed by bacterial infections, which in turn could lead to bumble foot due to penetration of 'a strange body'. However, we also saw foot wounds in hens on dry litter. Perhaps the wet conditions of the free-range area added to the foot problems or it was caused by perch design in these hens as was found by Tauson and Abrahamsson [40]. According to their results, both the rectangular and the round perches in our study did not meet the hens' needs.

4.9. Comb Color

The hybrid significantly explained the overall difference in comb color. Therefore, further calculations were only done for the most-used hybrid: H&N Silver Nick. FRU was related to darker combs. Flocks that were more fearful during our visits had lighter combs, but we could not find comparable results in the literature. Flocks that tested positively for one or more intestinal parasites tended to have darker combs. It is not clear whether this is a causal relation, because comb color in free-living red grouse is lighter in birds infected with internal parasites [41]. Spending more time in the free-range area is related to darker combs. A comparable finding is reported by Whay *et al.* [42].

5. Conclusions

With a mean flock size of 9,300 hens and 107 farms in 2008, the organic poultry sector has shown that it is able to become a serious alternative for existing intensive animal production. The presence of a free-range area is the most characteristic aspect of the organic system. Our study shows that a flock's welfare benefits from using this free-range area, as is shows less feather pecking damage if it uses it. Concerning the presence of feather pecking damage and thus animal welfare, the organic system has the potential to perform better than 'indoor' poultry husbandry systems because of the presence of the free range area. The organic flocks perform about the same or worse than other commercial systems for several other factors. Improvements are desirable for mortality, internal parasites, keel bone deformations, and foot sole lesions. However, it can be questioned whether these physical consequences can be attributed to the housing system or if they are the result of the interaction between genotype and environment. The organic system uses the same high productive (and perhaps thus vulnerable) genotypes as other commercial systems in an environment that is still artificial.

Acknowledgments

The authors gratefully thank and acknowledge the funding by the Dutch Ministry of Economic Affairs for project 'Relation between farm factors and animal health', BO-04-002-004.015.

Author Contributions

Both authors contributed to the design of the study. Bestman did the farm visits. Wagenaar did the statistical analyses. Both authors wrote the article.

Conflict of Interest

The authors declare no conflict of interest.

References and Notes

1. Bestman, M. Keeping Chickens without Feather Pecking (in Dutch); Louis Bolk Institute: Driebergen, The Netherlands, 2002; p. 17.
2. Agricultural Database Dutch National Statistic Institute (CBS). Available online: http://statline.cbs.nl/StatWeb/publication/?VW=T&DM=SLNL&PA=81517NED&D1=a&D2=a& D3=l&HD=120309–1138&HDR=G2,G1&STB=T (accessed on 27 February 2013).
3 Regulation Organic Animal Husbandry. Available online: http://www.skal.nl/LinkClick.aspx? fileticket=an0aCY%2b7kWE%3d&tabid=108&language=nl-NL (accessed on 27 February 2013).
4. Fiks-van Niekerk, T.; Reuvekamp, B.; Landman, W. Monitoring of Organic Farms. More Infections as on Cage Farms (in Dutch). *Pluimveehouderij* **2003**, *33*, 10–11.
5. Lampkin, N. *Organic Poultry Production*; Report to MAFF; Welsh Institute of Rural Studies, University of Wales: Aberystwyth, UK, 1997.
6. Keutgen, H.; Wurm, S.; Ueberschär, S. Pathologisch-anatomische Untersuchungen bei Legehennen aus Verschiedenen Haltungssystemen. *Deutsche Tierärztliche Wochenschrift.* **1999**, *106*, 127–133.
7. Berg, C. Health and Welfare in Organic Poultry Production. *Acta Vet. Scand.* **2001**, *S95*, 37–45.
8. Sommer, F. A Decade of Experience with Free-Range Poultry Farming in Austria. Is This the Future? In Proceedings of the 50th Western Poultry Disease Conference, Davis, CA, USA, 24–26 March 2001; pp. 95–96.
9. Hegelund, L.; Soerensen, J.T.; Hermansen, J.E. Welfare and Productivity of Laying Hens in Commercial Organic Egg Production Systems in Denmark. *NJAS* **2006**, *54*, 147–155.
10. Tauson, R.; Kjaer, J.; Maria, G.A.; Cepero, R.; Holm, K.-E. Applied Scoring of Integument and Health in Laying Hens. *Anim. Sci. Pap. Rep.* **2005**, *23*(Suppl 1), 153–159; and references therein.

11. Vestergaard, K.S.; Kruijt, J.P.; Hogan, J.A. Feather Pecking and Chronic Fear in Groups of Red Jungle Fowl: Their Relations to Dustbathing, Rearing Environment and Social Status. *Anim. Behav.* **1993**, *45*, 1127–1140.

12. El-Lethey, H.; Aerni, V.; Jungi, T.W.; Wechsler, B. Stress and Feather Pecking in Laying Hens in Relation to Housing Conditions. *Brit. Poultry Sci.* **2000**, *41*, 22–28.

13. Gentle, M.J.; Hunter, L.N. Physiological and Behavioural Responses Associated with Feather Removal in Gallus gallus var domesticus. *Res. Vet. Sci.* **1990**, *27*, 149–157.

14. Loefs, R. Organic Laying Hen Sector is Marking Time (in Dutch). *Pluimveehouderij* **2008**, *38*, 50–51.

15. Fossum, O.; Jansson, D.S.; Etterlin, P.E.; Vagsholm, I. Causes of Mortality in Laying Hens in Different Housing Systems in 2001 to 2004. *Acta Vet. Scand.* **2009**, *51*.

16. Sherwin, C.M.; Richards, G.J.; Nicol, C.J. Comparison of the Welfare of Layer Hens in 4 housing systems in the UK. *Brit. Poultry Sci.* **2010**, *51*, 488–499.

17. Stahl, P.; Ruette, S.; Groset, L. Predation on Free-ranging Poultry by Mammalian and Avian Predators: Field Loss Estimates in a French Rural Area. *Mammal Rev.* **2002**, *32*, 227–234.

18. Häne, M.; Huber-Eicher, B.; Fröhlich, E. Survey of Laying Hen Husbandry in Switzerland. *World's Poultry Sci. J.* **2000**, *56*, 21–31.

19. Moberly, R.I.; White, P.C.L.; Harris, S. Mortality due to Fox Predation in Free-range Poultry Flocks in Britain. *Vet. Rec.* **2004**, *155*, 48–52.

20. Bestman, M.W.P.; Wagenaar, J. Farm Level Factors Associated with Feather Pecking Damage in Organic Laying Hens. *Livest. Prod. Sci.* **2003**, *80*, 133–140.

21. Green, L.E.; Lewis, K.; Kimpton, A.; Nicol, C.J. A Cross Sectional Study of the Prevalence of Feather Pecking Damage in Laying Hens in Alternative Systems and its Association with Management and Disease. *Vet. Rec.* **2000**, *147*, 233–238.

22. Mahboub, H.D.H.; Müller, J.; von Borell, E. Outdoor Use, Tonic Immobility, Heterophil/lymphocyte Ratio and Feather Condition in Free-range Laying Hens of Different Genotype. *Brit. Poultry Sci.* **2004**, *45*, 738–744.

23. Nicol, C.J.; Pötzsch, C.; Lewis, K.; Green, L.E. Matched Concurrent Case-control Study of Risk Factors for Feather Pecking Damage in Hens on Free-range Commercial Farms in the UK. *Brit. Poultry Sci.* **2003**, *44*, 515–523.

24. van Krimpen, M.; Binnendijk, G.P.; van den Anker, I.; Heetkamp, M.J.W.; Kwakkel, R.P.; van den Brand, H. Effects of Ambient Temperature, Plumage Condition and Housing System on Energy Partitioning and Performance in Laying Hens, thereby Predicting Energy Intake. **2014**, in preparation.

25. Lay, D.C.; Fulton, R.M.; Hester, P.Y.; Karcher, D.M.; Kjaer, J.B.; Mench, J.A.; Mullens, B.A.; Newberry, R.C.; Nicol, C.J.; O'Sullivan, N.P.; Porter, R.E. Hen Welfare in Different Housing Systems. *Poultry Sci.* **2011**, *90*, 278–294.

26. Thamsborg, S.M.; Roepstorff, A.; Larsen, M. Integrated and Biological Control of Parasites in Organic and Conventional Production Systems. *Vet. Parasitol.* **1999**, *84*, 169–186.

27. Poultry parasites. Available online: http://www.gddeventer.com/pluimvee/zoekresultaat?search= wormen (accessed on 27 February 2013).

28. Huber-Eicher, B. A Survey of Layer-type Pullet Rearing in Switzerland. *World's Poultry Sci. J.* **1999**, *55*, 83–91.

29. Blokhuis, H.J.; van der Haar, J.W. Effects of Pecking Incentives during Rearing on Feather Pecking of Laying Hens. *Brit. Poultry Sci.* **1992**, *33*, 17–24.

30. Wechsler, B.; Huber-Eicher, B. The Effect of Foraging Material and Perch Height on Feather Pecking and Feather Damage in Laying Hens. *Appl. Anim. Behav. Sci.* **1998**, *58*, 131–141.

31. Nicol, C.J.; Gregory, N.G.; Knowles, T.G.; Parkman, I.D.; Wilkins, L.J.; Differential Effects of Increased Stocking Density, Mediated by Increased Flock Size, on Feather Pecking and Aggression in Laying Hens. *Appl. Anim. Behav. Sci.* **1999**, *65*, 137–152.

32. Savory, C.J.; Mann, J.S.; Macleod, M.G. Incidence of Pecking Damage in Growing Bantams in Relation to Food Form, Group Size, Stocking Density, Dietary Tryptophan Concentrations and Dietary Protein Source. *Brit. Poultry Sci.* **1999**, *40*, 579–584.

33. Huber-Eicher, B.; Audigé, L. Analysis of Risk Factors for the Occurrence of Feather Pecking in Laying Hen Growers. *Brit. Poultry Sci.* **1999**, *40*, 599–604.

34. Hüber-Eicher, B.; Sebö, F. The Prevalence of Feather Pecking Damage and Development in Commercial Flocks of Laying Hens. *Appl. Anim. Behav. Sci.* **2001**, *74*, 223–231.

35. Pötzsch, C.J.; Lewis, K.; Nicol, C.J.; Green, L.E. A Cross-sectional Study of the Prevalence of Vent Pecking in Laying Hens in Alternative Systems and its Associations with Feather Pecking Damage, Management and Disease. *Appl. Anim. Behav. Sci.* **2001**, *74*, 259–272.

36. Lambton, S.L.; Knowles, T.G.; Yorke, C.; Nicol, C.J. Risk Factors Affecting the Development of Vent Pecking and Cannibalism in Loose Housed Laying Hen Flocks. In Proceedings of the Poultry Welfare Symposium, Cervia, Italy, 18–22 May 2009; p. 13.

37. Wilkins, L.J.; McKinstry, J.L.; Avery, N.C.; Knowles, T.G.; Brown, S.N.; Tarlton, J.; Nicol, C.J. Influence of Housing System and Design on Bone Strength and Keel Bone Fractures in Laying Hens. *Vet. Rec.* **2011**, *169*, 414–420.

38. Gregory, N.G.; Wilkins, L.J. Effect of Age on Bone Strength and the Prevalence of Broken Bones in Perchery Laying Hens. *N. Z. Vet. J.* **1995**, *44*, 31–32.

39. Nicol, C.J.; Brown, S.N.; Glen, E.; Pope, S.J.; Short, F.J.; Warriss, P.D.; Zimmerman, P.H.; Wilkins, L.J. Effects of Stocking Density, Flock Size and Management on the Welfare of Laying Hens in Single-tier Aviaries. *Brit. Poul. Sci.* **2006**, *47*, 135–146.

40. Tauson, R.; Abrahamsson, P. Foot and Skeletal Disorders in Laying Hens. Effects of Perch Design, Hybrid, Housing System and Stocking Density. *Acta Agr. Scand.* **1994**, *44*, 110–119.

41. Mougeot, F.; Martínez-Padilla, J.; Bortolotti, J.; Webster, L.M.I.; Piertney, S.B. Physiological Stress Links Parasites to Carotenoid-based Color Signals. *J. Evol. Biol.* **2010**, *23*, 643–650.

42. Whay, H.R.; Main, D.C.J.; Green, L.E.; Heaven, G.; Howell, H.; Morgan, M.; Pearson, A.; Webster, A.J.F. Assessment of the Behaviour and Welfare of Laying Hens on Free-range units. *Vet. Rec.* **2007**, *161*, 119–128.

5

Assessing Food Preferences in Dogs and Cats: A Review of the Current Methods

Christelle Tobie *, Franck Péron and Claire Larose

SPF Diana, ZA du Gohélis, Elven 56250, France; E-Mails: fperon@diana-petfood.com (F.P.); cforges@diana-petfood.com (C.L.)

* Author to whom correspondence should be addressed; E-Mail: ctobie@diana-petfood.com.

Academic Editor: Edgar Chambers IV

Simple Summary: The objective of this review is to present the different approaches and techniques used to assess petfood palatability, either with expert panels or naïve individuals (in-home panels).

Abstract: Food is a major aspect of pet care; therefore, ensuring that pet foods are not only healthful but attractive to companion animals and their owners is essential. The petfood market remains active and requires ongoing evaluation of the adaptation and efficiency of the new products. Palatability—foods' characteristics enticing animals and leading them to consumption—is therefore a key element to look at. Based on the type of information needed, different pet populations (expert or naïve) can be tested to access their preference and acceptance for different food products. Classical techniques are the one-bowl and two-bowl tests, but complementary (*i.e.*, operant conditioning) and novel (*i.e.*, exploratory behavior) approaches are available to gather more information on the evaluation of petfood palatability.

Keywords: pet food; palatability; acceptance; preference; dogs; cats; emotional palatability; pet parenting; cognition

1. Introduction

The petfood market remains active and dynamic. Recent data revealed a constant increase in the pet population reaching 3.5 billion dogs and cats worldwide in 2014 [1]. In parallel, pet food sales are increasing even faster reaching 131.7 billion euro [2] over the same period. The petfood industries are regularly innovating and developing new products/formulas. Between January 2013 and October 2014 more than 4000 snack and 6000 food products (3000 dry and 3200 wet pet foods [3]) were launched on the market worldwide.

When developing new products, the petfood industries have to find a compromise between nutritional quality and palatability, particularly for diets claiming health benefits such as obesity or diabetes management. Even the best formulated diets can be inefficient or not popular among pet owners if the animal refuses to eat it. Palatability is consequently a crucial attribute for pet foods.

The hedonic properties of food are often defined by an attractive taste and are understood not only through the sensory characterization of food, such as smell, taste and mouthfeel but also through the nutritional and physiological post-ingestion effects. Palatability is related to how readily a food is accepted and measured in terms of its attractiveness and consumption. Because understanding animals' preference is not obvious, indirect objective methodologies have to be developed in order to rank different products based on animal feeding behaviors and reactions. Assessment of palatability in companion animals is strategic for developing foods, treats and (oral) medications that they will consume.

Domestic dogs and cats have different nutritional requirements [4], feeding behaviors [5,6] and are sensitive to numerous palatability drivers [7]. The sensory analysis of diets by pets is mostly based on preference and/or acceptance tests [8]. Such trials can be performed in in-home panels of naïve pets and in expert panels of animals trained to discriminate foods with different nutritional and sensory properties since they were young. In preference testing, animals have the choice between two different diets presented simultaneously whereas in the acceptability tests, only one type of food product is available. To enrich the classical palatability measurements, new methods and criteria have been developed focusing on selected animal behaviors proven to reflect in an innovative way, pet foods' palatability performance.

Feeding pets or giving them treats is a key moment which strengthens the bond between the owners and their animals. Referring to emotions and perceived palatability, recent protocol developments also took in consideration owners' perception of their pets' feeding enjoyment and consequently their perception of a diet's palatability. The important point is that all these palatability measurement methods are complementary; they can be combined to finally deliver an exhaustive evaluation of pet foods' overall palatability and performance.

In this review, the pros and cons of the different classical methods to assess petfood palatability are presented as well as newly developed and complementary techniques.

2. Panels and Methods Classically Used to Assess Food Preference and Acceptability

Palatability assessment tests can be run on two types of animal panels: either in pet centers with expert panels or in an in-home environment with owner's pets. Both approaches have advantages and constraints [9]. During the product development stage, the scientific and technical questions will lead towards one or the other option. Expert panels perform palatability tests on a daily basis. They can be specialized on one type of food (dry only or wet only) or test different types of diets with transition periods between each. The expert pets are more reliable and accurate than in-home pets, but need intensive training to be exposed to a diversity of foods; qualification tests when one product is known to be highly palatable compared to the other or when products are known to be equal to check that animals select as expected; and a permanent quality follow up to check their accuracy in discrimination, reproducibility of answers, and potential lateralization [10].

Quality tests should be conducted regularly in expert panels to control for any side bias. In this type of test, the animals are offered the same food and the expected outcome is to observe no significant difference (see Figure 1).

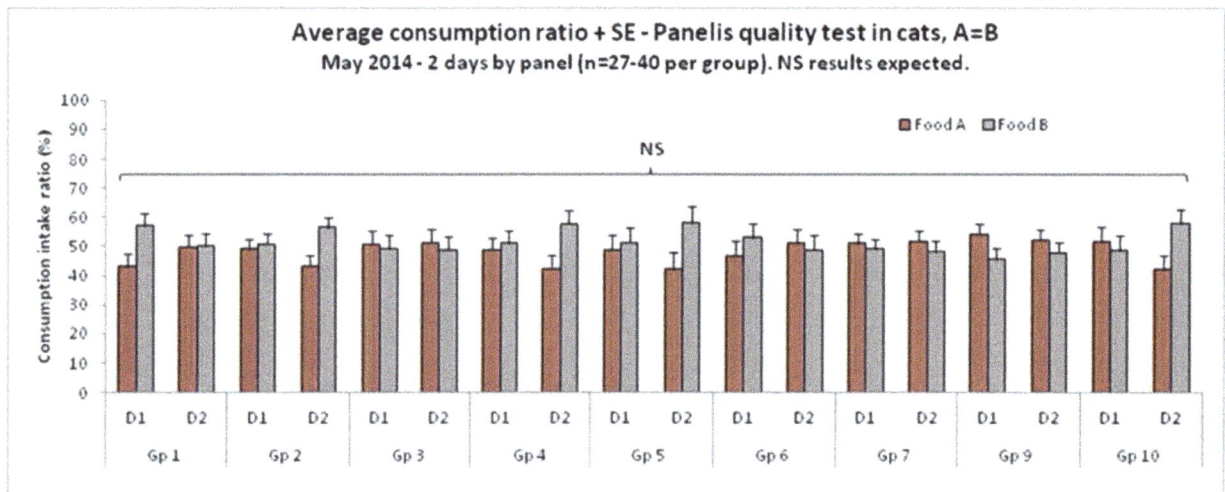

Figure 1. Average consumption ratio and Panelis quality test in cats, A = B, May 2014, 2 days by panel (*n* = 27–40 per group). None significant (NS) results expected.

The repeatability of testing conditions and the control of environmental perturbations are also among the key-characteristics of expert panels. To build such supervised "samples" of expert animals and to analyze this type of data (bimodal distribution), a minimum number of 30 individuals is necessary to secure statistical robustness. This level of requirements and control, on the dietary past for example, are necessary to limit the impact of biases (novelty effect, panel effect, *etc.*) on answers and obtain significant results even on finer differences [10]. In order to secure the reliability and relevancy of results, palatability assessment should also be performed on pets of varied ages, sizes and breeds, in good veterinary conditions and even more, on pets undergoing no stress.

In-home panels are constituted of family-owned pets that are selected according to different criteria (age, sex, dietary history, *etc.*). These tasters are naïve and do not have any training. They also have a lower testing frequency than expert panels and testing conditions are less controlled. In comparison with expert panels in-home pets feeding history can be vague and can lack diversity. It is very difficult to make sure that the testing protocol has been respected and that the owners' perceptions have not biased objective measurements. For all these reasons, palatability tests performed in such panels should include a lot more animals: ideally ≈100. The automation of the data collection can also provide additional reliability for the quantitative data gathered [11]. On the other hand, the main advantage of an in-home panel is in providing data representative of the final market: to get "real-life" feedback. Furthermore it is a good way to evaluate owners' reactions to the products' cosmetics and about their perception of palatability through pet-centric criteria.

The comparison between in-home and expert panel results often reveals differences, more or less important according to the type of product tested. Semi-expert panels consist in in-home dogs and cats trained and qualified to perform preference tests. For example, two-bowl tests performed on expert, semi-expert and in-home panels comparing different commercial dog dry foods showed that the outcome and conclusion could vary according to the panel used (see Figure 2).

Comparison between dog panels, January 2013 - 2 days by panel
Average Ratio + SE- Study conducted by SPF

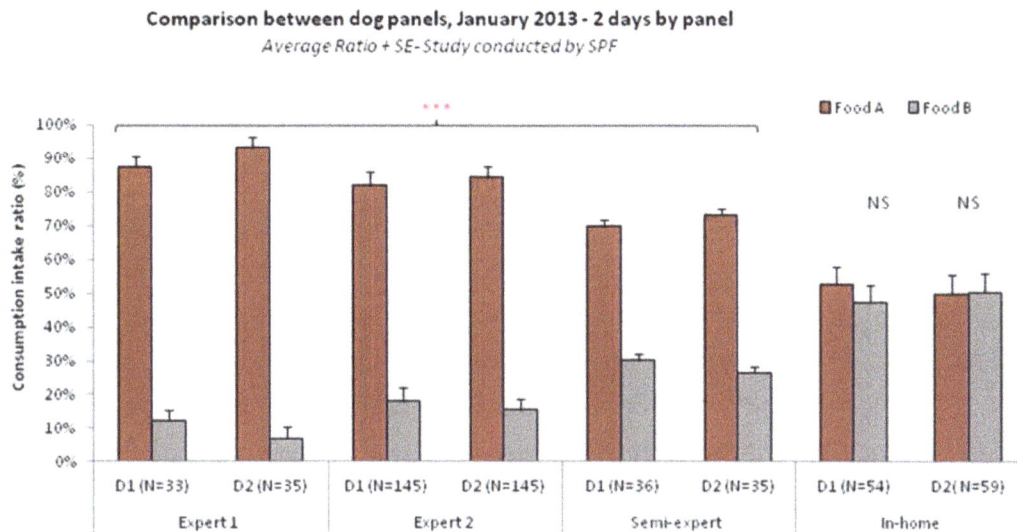

Figure 2. Comparison between dog panels, January 2013, 2 days by panel. Average Ratio + SE, Study conducted by Diana Pet Food.

For example in their study, Griffin *et al.* [9] found more consistency between the different panels when testing wet products. It was also noted that in-home panels may be more stable in their preferences [9] but that expert panels may be better discriminating small differences. Such discrepancies can be explained by all the factors we have just listed, related to pets' level of training, to their feeding history and to the testing environment.

Referring to the testing protocols, different approaches can be used in order to assess palatability differences between pet foods. In general all classical methods are based on the amount of each food consumed during a definite period. Two protocols are most commonly used. Preference testing is based on a simultaneous presentation of two diets, in order to measure if a preference is expressed by pets through quantities eaten of each product. Acceptance testing consists in the presentation of one diet only and in the assessment of the quantity eaten, as the expression of the product's intrinsic palatability. The food can be available for a limited period (for dogs for example) or for a longer period or even *ad libitum* to reproduce the "natural" conditions encountered in the home environment or, to respect a more natural feeding rhythm, for cats particularly.

The two-bowl test (or paired stimulus or *versus* test) compares how much of two foods, presented simultaneously, is eaten in a defined period of time. This is the most common test used in expert panels for dog and cat palatability assessment studies. It compares two products and establishes a preference based on the difference of quantities consumed. Waterhouse and Fritsch [12] and Hegsted *et al.* [13] described the general method and the possible factors that could influence the results. In such tests, two identical bowls are delivered simultaneously to the tested animal, each bowl containing one of the two products to be tested (A or B). The animal has free access to the bowls for a preset period of time. The quantity available in each bowl is more than sufficient to cover the energetic requirements. In general, the test is conducted in individual enclosures to avoid any social interactions or competition. At the end of the feeding time or when one bowl is finished, bowls are taken back and weighted again to measure the quantity consumed. For each pair of products tested a second test maybe necessary, this time switching their relative position, in order to control any position bias. This second measure enables an evaluation of repeatability.

Important parameters in this two-pan test include the first choice that is the first food product tasted, reflecting the olfactory perception and attractiveness; the amount of food consumed; the ratio (A/B) of food consumed; the percentage of food intake (A/(A+B)) [14] and the preference ratio (quantity of food A consumed over the total of food distributed). Usually the percentage of consumption is used [15]. The two-pan test enables a ranking between different products but is not transitive as the "preference" is based on a forced choice. The palatability of the diet is not considered *per se* but in comparison to the other diet, which means that all the paired comparisons should be tested.

Some *versus* trials are conducted with pets in-home [11], but it is generally less precise in this condition due to the lack of environment control (for example greedy dogs finishing both bowls if the owner did not remove them early, or several cats sharing the same bowl, *etc.*). Thus, it is preferable that the two-bowl tests be conducted using expert panels as they allow control of the possible bias [10,12,16].

One inconvenience of two-pan testing is that the method does not offer control of how different foods (smell and taste) may affect the palatability of each other or of the long-term effects of caloric and nutritional value. This technique may also lead to animals consuming excessive quantities of food, if necessary human resources are not available to remove bowls when one is finished, or enough food from both bowls is consumed.

The one-bowl test (or one-pan, or single stimulus, or monadic test) [17], in which the animal has free access to a single food for a determined amount of time, is used to measure only the acceptability of a food product. This method is quite similar to the situation that can be found at home where a pet-owner introduces a new food product [18] and, thus, is well adapted to in-home panels. The indicators of this kind of testing will be mostly the quantity consumed and sometimes the speed of consumption. Furthermore, when tested in-home, it is possible to use questionnaires in order to enrich the information gathered. For example, additional data such as human perceptions of the food [19] or the animals' enthusiasm to eat it [11,20] can be collected. Thus, owners can provide not only information about home environment and dietary history of their animal but also their impressions on the different diets and report any behavior or physiological modifications.

Several factors can influence the results of the one-bowl test such as the seasonal effect (*i.e.*, in cats: eating less during winter [21]) or a daily variation (*i.e.*, dog eating more during their afternoon meal compared to the morning meal; personal communication) requiring a calculation of a reference consumption level and adapted distributed ration that would take into account those factors. This is particularly important as the interpretation of the "unique" value delivered may sometimes be complex.

3. Complementary Methods and New Approaches

It is possible to implement complementary indicators and provide additional information to classical preference and acceptance tests.

3.1. Liking Test

The Liking test consists of a one-bowl test with adjusted food quantities, which enables the animal to finish the bowl infrequently, and available for a preset period of time [22]. The monitored indicators reflect meaningful criteria for owners in the understanding of their pets' feeding enjoyment: the percentage of finished bowls and refusals; the consumption speed; and the gap with the reference consumption rate (RCR) of each individual (see Figure 3). The RCR consists of the ratio between the individual level of consumption at the test and the individual reference consumption based on its food intake history and other natural variations (season, meal of the day, *etc.*). The analysis of the deviation is reported for the all panel. If the difference is significant and negative: individuals of the panel did not like the food (or at least eat less than usual) and on the contrary if the difference is significant and positive, individuals enjoyed their food.

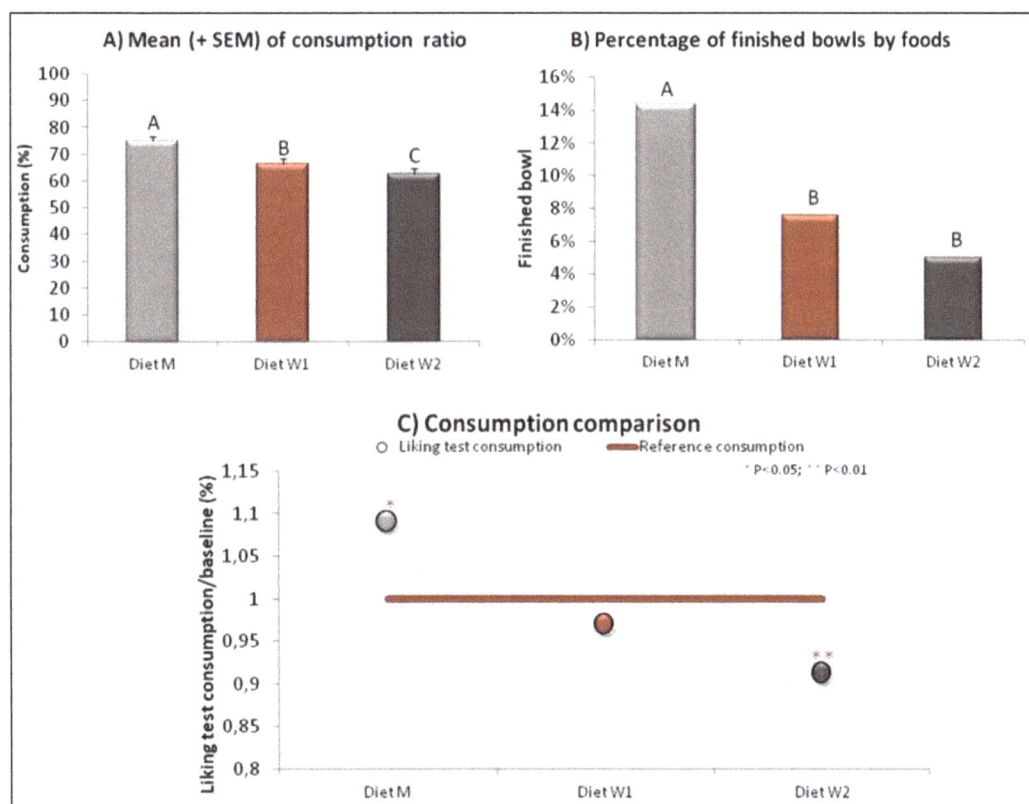

Figure 3. Evaluation of diets M, W1 and W2 by a Liking test conducted on an expert panel (*n* = 38, Panelis) (**A**) consumption ratio, (**B**) finished bowls and (**C**) consumption of the diets expressed relative to a reference consumption. Differing letters identify significant differences between the products.

This one-bowl test is run with expert panels as it was developed to provide higher accuracy and reliability thanks to the control of specific biases potentially impacting monadic testing at home. It is even possible to rank different products tested with monadic tests but some parameters should be adapted, such as the randomization of the order of the different food products presented across the tested population and specific statistical treatment. A mixed model is used to analyze the differences between groups' means on fixed variables. A random variable is used to take into account the individual variability and to extrapolate the results to a larger population.

3.2. Kinetics

Fine-grained measurement is the cumulative amount eaten on a moment-by-moment basis during the test used both for one-bowl and two-bowl tests. This approach can provide quantitative information about individual feeding styles (rapid eaters *vs.* slow eaters), the way animals distribute their feeding between two foods in a choice test and, in some cases, the initial disruptive effects of a new diet [18]. Using the one-bowl method on a preset period of 20 h with a follow up of the quantity consumed helps to compare the profile of acceptance of the different products [23], which did not distinguish one from the other during the preference test. Kinetics can be used to measure new indicators of performance and enjoyment, including criteria reflecting attractiveness: average time before the first visit (passage or feeding events), average consumption per feeding events, number of passage without consumption, *etc.* (see Figure 4).

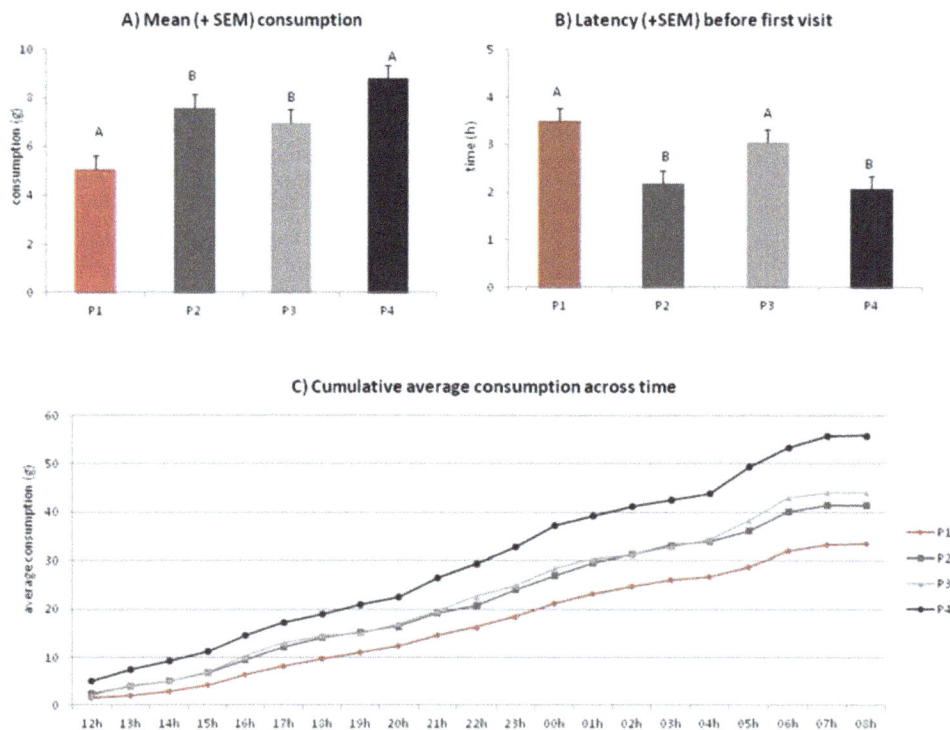

Figure 4. Four dry cat foods, differing only by the composition of the palatability enhancer applied in coating, were evaluated in sequential monadic conditions by a 40 cats expert panel (Panelis). Individual data such as time and quantities eaten were recorded automatically during a 20 h period. (**A**) average consumption per passage (adjusted mean +SEM); (**B**) average time before the first visit (adjusted mean + SEM); and (**C**) cumulative average consumption across time. Differing letters identify significant differences between the products ($p < 0.05$).

This tool enables to differentiate between an immediate attractiveness and its evolution across time. It is also adapted to the observation of feeding behaviors in front of specific diets: individuals—cats particularly- are supposed to reduce their number of visits to the bowl and/or meal size when fed with a "satiety" product compared to a standard food product. At the end of the feeding period we may observe diets consumed in different quantities, the consumption rate of the "satiety" product being slower. Even over a medium-term food intake study, dogs showed a difference in their feeding pattern with a satiety effect more pronounced for the high-protein high-fiber diet compared to the high-protein low-fiber diet, with both diets having equivalent palatability [24].

In preference testing (two-bowl test) and in acceptability testing (one-bowl test) the animal performing the test may not have other food choices than the one presented, and may be forced to eat a food even if they find it less palatable. Furthermore the post ingestion effects can impact on the expression of a preference, for instance, when testing weight management diets where it would be difficult to distinguish enhanced efficacy and reduced palatability. Complementary methods can be used looking not only at the quantity eaten but also at the "value" of the food when use as a reward in a learning task.

3.3. Concurrent Schedule Paradigm (CSP)

The concurrent schedule paradigm or operant conditioning is a procedure used to assess the strength of an animal's motivation to eat [25]. This method used to compare quantitative and qualitative differences (quantify the hedonic value of foods) requires a specific motor action directed to specifically designed device such as a lever-pressing apparatus [25,26] or through human-animal interaction (e.g., nose-touching on experimenter's hand; [27]). This kind of approach assesses animal's reactivity to food with minimum post-ingestion complications (relatively small food quantity) and enables comparison of very different food products as it is the "currency" (i.e., motivation to press the lever) that is compared. Technically demanding as it may requires a specific device and software and time consuming, the CSP requires highly trained individuals, tested over a relatively long period.

3.4. Cognitive Palatability Assessment Protocol (CPAP)

Araujo and Milgram [28] developed a method based on associative learning consisting in an object discrimination learning task where the animal can express a preference without any food intake. The dog can interact with three different objects, two of them paired with different types of food. Once the animal develops a preference for a specific object and its associated outcome, the pairs are switched and the dog has to learn the new association if he wants to keep receiving its "preferred" food product. The no reward object provides a control for individuals without any preference between the two compared foods. This preference testing approach can vary to examine short- or long-term preferences without confounding nutritional or caloric effects. While comparing the CPAP with the two-pan tests, the authors found that it was possible to compare different types of products (moist vs. dry for instance); that the differences between the products were stronger even with small sample size; and that the preference was stable across time and repetitions [29]. The results suggest that the CPAP is less sensitive to the effects of prior feeding and satiation than the two-bowl test [29]. This method also requires extensive training and more time but at the same time fewer individuals are necessary to obtain significant reliable data. The CPAP seems less adapted to cats as it requests sustained attention from the tested individual.

Concurrent schedule paradigm and CPAP methods may not be biologically relevant as they are very different from the real living conditions and feeding habits of the pets.

3.5. Exploratory Behavior

A previous experiment looked at the cat body language and behavior within a context of feeding period, with wet food, and found differences related to palatability [30]: licking or sniffing the food bowl and lip licking were associated with palatable food products whereas sniffing the food or nose licking reflected some aversion for the product. However, a similar study conducted on dry food did not reveal any difference (Personal communication). More recent studies assess differences in the perceived palatability of products using a spontaneous behavior: the olfactory exploration. The role of olfaction at feeding time is multiple [31]: to locate the food source—that may be less relevant for domestic species; to assess the food organoleptic aspects, toxicity, *etc.*; and to stimulate the gut secretion. Other studies have looked at the spontaneous behavior of the pets when facing different food products either presented sequentially (one-bowl test) or simultaneously (two-bowl test). In the Becques *et al.* [32] study for instance, the cats were video recorded during their feedings over several days. Behaviors and postures were coded according to different categories and correlated with food intake measures. In the dog study [33] individuals first had the opportunity to taste the different food products before experiencing the situation where a wire mesh was impeding the access to the different bowls. The authors looked at the time spent exploring both food locations. The results revealed that cats [32] spent significantly longer sniffing at the product less preferred. Dogs were the opposite [33] exploring longer the preferred food product. The difference between the two species could be explained by their natural history and dietary behavior [5,6] or by the difference in the protocol used, as cats could access the food product at the end, while dogs could not.

4. Conclusions

During the past 30 years, the same classical tests and criteria have been mostly used to assess pet food palatability. Only recently new approaches and complementary indicators have been developed in order to provide more information and enrich palatability measurement. Analyzed consumption parameters are no longer exclusively intake ratios, and new approaches are no longer exclusively focused on organoleptic and nutritional orientations; they are now considering the emotional dimension of palatability performance. New assessments integrate the triangular relationship in petfooding, considering not only the behavioral expressions of pets but also the interactions with their owners and finally the owners' perception of their pet enjoyment.

Each of the methods counts advantages and disadvantages, but according to the type of questions, to the targets and the panel resources available, it is possible to select one or another method and sometimes even a combination of several. All the palatability measurement methods are complementary, can be combined and finally deliver an in-depth evaluation of pet foods' comprehensive palatability and performance (see Table 1).

Table 1. Summary of the pros and cons of the different methods.

	⊕ WHAT FOR	⊖ LIMITS	⊕ WHAT ELSE
TWO-BOWL TESTS	• New products in development • Measurement of fine differences (ingredient effects on same kibble base, screening of new formulas) • Rather on expert panels	• Forced comparison in expert panel ≠ in-home • Not adapted to compare different nutritional values	• CPAP to remove the influence of food intake • Kinetics to differentiate palatability levels with new criteria and visualize how preference has been built
ONE-PAN TESTS	ON EXPERT PANELS: • Product development validation • Measurement of product acceptability in natural conditions, of specific criteria related to enjoyment observation or to nutritional specificities such as weight management . . . • Comparison of expected bigger differences ON IN-HOME PANELS: • Access to owners perception	• Lack of accuracy due to uncontrolled parameters • Possible subjective interpretation of owners	• Kinetics to differentiate iso palatable products with new criteria or analyze consumption of different nutritional values or physiological effects • Liking tests for new enjoyment and behavioral criteria

Acknowledgments

We would like to thanks Laure Le Paih for the graphs, Laura Clover and Stan Wrobel for their help improving the manuscript.

Author Contributions

The manuscript was composed by Christelle Tobie and Franck Péron and reviewed by Claire Larose.

Conflicts of Interest

All the authors are employees of Diana Pet Food, a company that provides palatability testing to the pet food industry.

References

1. Euromonitor International. Pet population. Pet Care. 2015. Available online: http://www.euromonitor.com/pet-care (accessed on 28 October 2014).
2. Euromonitor International. Market sizes. Pet Care. 2015. Available online: http://www.euromonitor.com/pet-care (accessed on 28 October 2014).
3. Mintel GNPD. 2014. Available online: http://www.mintel.com/global-new-products-database (accessed on 28 October 2014).

4. National Research Council. *Nutrient Requirements of Dogs and Cats*; National Academy Press: Washington, DC, USA, 2006.

5. Bourgeois, H.; Elliot, D.; Marniquet, P.; Soulard, Y. Dietary behavior of dogs and cats. *Bulletin de l'Académie Vétérinaire de France* **2006**, *4*, 301–308.

6. Bradshaw, J.W. The evolutionary basis for the feeding behavior of domestic dogs (*Canis familiaris*) and cats (*Felis catus*). *J. Nutr.* **2006**, *136*, 1927–1931.

7. Fournier, M.; de Ratuld, A.; Callejon, L. Cats and Dogs Palatability Drivers. *Animals*, submitted.

8. Koppel, K. Sensory analysis of pet foods. *J. Sci. Food Agri.* **2014**, *11*, 2148–2153.

9. Griffin, R.W.; Scott, G.C.; Cante, C.J. Food preferences of dogs housed in testing-kennels and in consumers' homes: Some comparisons. *Neurosci. Biobehavioral Rev.* **1984**, *8*, 253–259.

10. Larose, C. Criteria to assure reliability of palatability tests. *PETS Int. Mag.* **2003**, *August*, 14–15.

11. Vondran, J.C. A Two Pan Feeding Trial with Companion Dogs: Considerations for Future Testing. Master Thesis, Kansas State University, Manhattan, KS, USA, 2013.

12. Waterhouse, H.N.; Fritsch, C.W. Dog Food Palatability Tests and Sources of Potential Bias. *Lab. Anim. Care* **1967**, *17*, 93–102.

13. Gershoff, S.; Hegsted, D.; Lentini, E. The development of palatability tests for cats. *Am. J. Vet. Res.* **1956**, *17*, 733–737.

14. Shi, Z. Palatability, a critical component of pet foods. *Feed Tech.* **2000**, *4*, 34–37.

15. Griffin, R.W. Palatability testing, two-pan tests: Methods and data analysis techniques. *Petfood Ind.* **1996**, *Sept-Oct*, 4–6.

16. Larose, C. Bad habits: How to prevent petfood palatability test distortions. *Petfood Ind.* **2004**, *September*, 12–18.

17. Rashotte, M.E.; Foster, D.F.; Austin, T. Two-pan and operant lever-press tests of dogs' preference for various foods. *Neurosci. Biobehavioral. Rev.* **1984**, *8*, 231–237.

18. Smith, J.C.; Rashotte, M.E.; Austin, T.; Griffin, R.W. Fine-grained measures of dogs' eating behavior in single-pan and two-pan tests. *Neurosci. Biobehavioral. Rev.* **1984**, *8*, 243–251.

19. Di Donfrancesco, B.; Koppel, K.; Swaney-Stueve, M.; Chambers, E., IV. Consumer Acceptance of Dry Dog Food Variations. *Animals* **2014**, *4*, 313–330.

20. Sanderson, S.L.; Finco, D.R.; Pogrelis, A.D.; Stacy, L.M.; Unger, C.F. Owner impressions of three premium diets fed to healthy adult dogs. *J. Am. Vet. Med. Assoc.* **2005**, *227*, 1931–1936.

21. Serisier, S.; Feugier, A.; Delmotte, S.; Biourge, V.; German, A.J. Seasonal Variation in the Voluntary Food Intake of Domesticated Cats (*Felis Catus*). *PLOS ONE* **2014**, *9*, e96071.

22. Becques, A.; Roguès, J.; Nicéron, C. The liking test, bringing new dimensions to dog and food palatability measurment. In Proceedings of the 6th European Conference on Sensory and Consumer Research, Copenhagen, Denmark, 2014; p. 295.

23. Roguès, J.; le Paih, L.; Forges, C.; Niceron, C. Kinetics of consumption, an innovative tool to measure cat food palatability. In Proceedings of the 6th European Conference on Sensory and Consumer Research, Copenhagen, Denmark, 2014; p. 126.

24. Weber, M.; Bissot, T.; Servet, E.; Sergheraert, R.; Biourge, V.; German, A.J. A High-Protein, High-Fiber Diet Designed for Weight Loss Improves Satiety in Dogs. *J. Vet. Int. Med.* **2007**, *21*, 1203–1208.

25. Rashotte, M.E.; Smith, J.C. Operant conditioning methodology in the assessment of food preferences: introductory comments. *Neurosci. Biobehavioral Rev.* **1984**, *8*, 211–215.

26. Collier, G.; Johnson, D.F.; Morgan, C. Meal patterns of cats encountering variable food procurement costs. *J. Exp. Anal. Behav.* **1997**, *67*, 303–310.

27. Vicars, S.M.; Miguel, C.F.; Sobie, J.L. Assessing preference and reinforcer effectiveness in dogs. *Behav. Process.* **2014**, *103*, 75–83.

28. Araujo, J.A.; Milgram, N.W. A novel cognitive palatability assessment protocol for dogs. *J. Anim. Sci.* **2004**, *82*, 2200–2208.

29. Araujo, J.A.; Studzinski, C.M.; Larson, B.T.; Milgram, N.W. Comparison of the cognitive palatability assessment protocol and the two-pan test for use in assessing palatability of two similar foods in dogs. *Am. J. Vet. Res.* **2004**, *65*, 1490–1496.

30. Van den Bos, R.; Meijer, M.K.; Spruijt, B.M. Taste reactivity patterns in domestic cats (*Felis silvestris catus*). *Appl. Anim. Behav. Sci.* **2000**, *69*, 149–168.

31. Bradley, B.L. Animal flavor types and their specific uses in compounds feeds by species and age. In *Palatability Flavor Use Animal Feed*; Verlag Paul Parey: Berlin, Germany, 1980; pp. 110–122.

32. Becques, A.; Larose, C.; Baron, C.; Niceron, C.; Féron, C.; Gouat, P. Behaviour in order to evaluate the palatability of pet food in domestic cats. *App. Anim. Behav. Sci.* **2014**, *159*, 55–61.

33. Ellis, S.; Thompson, H.; Riemer, S.; Burman, O. Developing a novel method of assessing food preference in the domestic dog. In Proceedings 3rd Canine Science Forum, Lincoln, UK, 2014; p. 220.

6

Conscientious Objection to Harmful Animal Use within Veterinary and Other Biomedical Education

Andrew Knight

Ross University School of Veterinary Medicine, P.O. Box 334, Basseterre, St Kitts, West Indies;
E-Mail: aknight@rossvet.edu.kn;

Simple Summary: Classes in which animals are harmed are controversial within veterinary and other life and health sciences courses. Increasingly, students object to the harmful use of animals, and request humane teaching alternatives. Such cases can raise important animal welfare, legal and administrative concerns for universities. Several have implemented formal policies to guide their responses, maximising the likelihood of optimal and consistent outcomes. This paper reviews the development of these conscientious objection policies within Australian veterinary schools, and examines their underlying legal foundations. It concludes with recommendations for other universities considering how to respond to such cases.

Abstract: Laboratory classes in which animals are seriously harmed or killed, or which use cadavers or body parts from ethically debatable sources, are controversial within veterinary and other biomedical curricula. Along with the development of more humane teaching methods, this has increasingly led to objections to participation in harmful animal use. Such cases raise a host of issues of importance to universities, including those pertaining to curricular design and course accreditation, and compliance with applicable animal welfare and antidiscrimination legislation. Accordingly, after detailed investigation, some universities have implemented formal policies to guide faculty responses to such cases, and to ensure that decisions are consistent and defensible from legal and other policy perspectives. However, many other institutions have not yet done so, instead dealing with such cases on an *ad hoc* basis as they arise. Among other undesirable outcomes this can lead to insufficient student and faculty preparation, suboptimal and inconsistent responses, and greater likelihood of legal challenge. Accordingly, this paper provides pertinent information about the evolution of conscientious objection policies within Australian veterinary schools, and about the jurisprudential bases for conscientious objection within

Australia and the USA. It concludes with recommendations for the development and implementation of policy within this arena.

Keywords: veterinary education; veterinary curriculum; conscientious objection; humane teaching methods; 3Rs

1. Introduction

Within veterinary education many thousands of animals have been killed worldwide during attempts to demonstrate scientific principles within preclinical years, or to teach practical skills within the clinical components of courses. Animals have been killed and dissected to demonstrate anatomical principles. Living animals or organs taken from them have been subjected to invasive experiments in physiology, biochemistry, pharmacology and parasitology laboratories. In many countries the mainstay of veterinary surgical practical training has been the practice of surgical procedures on healthy animals, which have frequently been killed following the procedure. Additionally, students in veterinary, animal science or other courses have often been required to assist with husbandry procedures on farm animals, such as teeth clipping in piglets, and castration in several species. These are usually legally sanctioned procedures, but because they can cause substantial pain and are frequently conducted without analgesia, they cause serious concerns for many students. Similarly, students may be required to attend abattoirs, although their role is usually observational rather than participatory.

However, alternative teaching methodologies have continued to develop for many of these educational applications, and databases including thousands of them now exist (e.g., NORINA: http://oslovet.norecopa.no). Such methods include computer simulations, high quality videos, ethically-sourced cadavers obtained from animals that have died naturally or in accidents, or most commonly, been euthanized for medical reasons, anatomical specimens preserved in a variety of ways, models, mannequins and surgical simulators, non-invasive self-experimentation, and supervised clinical experiences [1–6]. Social attitudes toward more traditional teaching exercises in which animals are harmed have also evolved in recent years and decades, concurrent with changes in student demographics and backgrounds. These factors have led to increasing desires among both students and faculty for more humane teaching methods, which are not reliant on harmful animal use.

Such desires can be particularly strong in certain students, such as those with certain ethical, religious or other viewpoints or sensitivities. Unlike faculty members who have usually been immersed in veterinary school environments for much longer periods, students asked to seriously harm or kill animals during their education may well be confronting such issues for the first time. Indeed, for many it will actually be the first time they've been directly required to harm or kill an animal, to further their educational or career goals. For some students this may profoundly conflict with their personal ethics, and indeed, with the reasons they've chosen to embark on a veterinary degree in the first place.

However, faculty opposition to student requests for humane teaching methods has been common, and has sometimes resulted in conflict. Universities that refuse to provide alternatives for students can find themselves legally liable, and in some cases damages have resulted. In 1995 University of Colorado medical student Safia Rubaii sued her university for US$95,000 after failing physiology, because she refused to perform a compulsory experiment which required her to give a lethal injection to an anaesthetised dog. She was forced to retake physiology at the Creighton University School of Medicine in Nebraska, where harmful animal use was not required. Dr. Rubaii successfully graduated from her university in the same year she sued it. When upholding her legal claims, the court also required the university to provide alternatives to future students who might request them, and these terminal dog laboratories have since been entirely replaced by humane alternatives [7,8].

Considerable adverse publicity has sometimes resulted from such cases, when curricular animal killing and academic sanctions applied to conscientiously objecting students are publicised through the mass media. Such cases have the potential to significantly impact the reputations of universities, because of negative public viewpoints about the harming and killing of healthy animals within curricula, and also, because of negative viewpoints about the application of academic sanctions to students or others who object to such animal use. The potential for reputational damage resulting from such treatment of students was aptly illustrated by Rutgers University law professors Francione and Charlton in 1992, in their legal guidebook for such students and their lawyers, who commented in relation to such cases that, *"The conclusion that most people draw is an important and correct one: those who exploit nonhuman animals are often not reluctant to violate the civil rights of humans."* [9] (p. x).

Such cases raise several ethical, legal and administrative issues of importance to veterinary and other biomedical faculties in which animals are used, including but not limited to those relating to animal welfare standards, applicable animal welfare and civil rights legislation, curricular design and professional accreditation requirements, the efficacy of both traditional and alternative teaching methods, academic freedom, and the non-discriminatory treatment of students.

Accordingly, within the last decade or more, some veterinary schools and universities have reviewed these issues in some detail, following which they have implemented policies allowing and formalizing the process of student conscientious objection to animal use considered harmful or objectionable. These have been called 'conscientious objection' or 'student choice' policies, with the latter being more common in North America. A recent publication, for example, described the establishment of such a policy at the recently established University of Adelaide's School of Animal and Veterinary Sciences [10].

However, despite the introduction of such policies at several veterinary schools and universities within Australia, the US and elsewhere, very little has been published about the jurisprudential bases for student conscientious objection. Recommendations for the development of policy within this arena are similarly lacking. Instead veterinary schools have developed policy on an *ad hoc* basis, usually in response to a case or crisis in this area.

Accordingly, this paper provides pertinent information about the jurisprudential bases for student conscientious objection within Australia and the US, with some additional insights from international jurisdictions. It then describes the evolution of conscientious objection policies within Australian veterinary schools, and concludes with recommendations for the development and implementation of policy within this arena.

2. Definitions and Jurisprudential Bases for Conscientious Objection

2.1. Importance of Conscientious Objection within Democracies

Conscientious objection is generally considered to occupy a legitimate, and often legally protected, position within democratic societies. Within Australia for example, statutes making provision for conscientious objection include those pertaining to the vaccination of children, the participation of nurses in medical procedures, and attendance of voters at polling booths on days proscribed by their religion. Another example is provided by the Western Australian Equal Opportunity Act (1984) [11], which in some circumstances outlaws discrimination in education on the grounds of belief. The NSW Law Reform Commission Community Law Reform Program 6th Report *Conscientious Objection to Jury Service* [12], which examined this issue in detail, affirmed that,

"Australian governments have often stressed the importance in a democratic system of respect for individual conscience" (p. 27), and, *"It is fundamental to society that people should not be compelled to act against their consciences in the performance of civic duties except in matters of overriding importance or urgency such as a national emergency"* (p. 44).

This principle is also supported by Article 18 of the Universal Declaration of Human Rights, proclaimed by the General Assembly of the United Nations in 1948 [13], which asserts that,

"Everyone has the right to freedom of thought, conscience, and religion; this right includes freedom to change his religion or belief, and freedom, either alone or in community with others and in public or private, to manifest his religion or belief in teaching, practice, worship and observance."

Additional international human rights legislation and the laws of several countries, e.g., England, India, Italy, The Netherlands and the US, support the rights of students to conscientiously object to participating in activities that run counter to their beliefs [9,14]. In 1993, for example, the Italian Parliament enacted a law recognizing the right of conscientious objectors to refuse to participate in animal experimentation and dissection. Similarly, Dutch universities are required to provide alternatives to students who do not wish to participate in exercises that harm animals. Likewise, a growing list of US states have passed laws requiring public schools to notify students (and/or their parents) that they may use alternatives to dissection or invasive live animal exercises without penalty [14].

2.2. Claims of Financial or Administrative Burden

These examples illustrate the fundamental importance normally accorded by modern democratic societies to the right of an individual to act in accordance with their conscience or belief. The *"national emergency"* case mentioned above provides a rare example in which violating such a right is considered acceptable. With respect to a conscientiously held student belief against participating in certain forms of educational animal use, as Francione and Charlton describe in their legal text on this issue [9], purported financial or administrative difficulties are not normally considered a sufficient reason for an educational institution to deny this student right, and to instead require that the student participate in such animal use on penalty of academic sanction. An institution may legitimately embark on such a course only if it can demonstrate that the financial and administrative burdens incurred by complying with such a student request would be so great as to seriously jeopardise the continued operation of the university or school—which could be contrary to the national interest.

However, although a body of relevant case law exists from the US and several other countries [9] this author is unaware of any cases in which such an argument has been successfully raised in a legal setting. This is hardly surprising, because humane teaching methods are often cheaper than methods that rely on harmful animal use. Indeed, economic factors have been one of the most important forces driving the introduction of humane teaching methods internationally. Educational animal use is rarely cheap, after all: the purchase, transportation, housing, feeding, veterinary care when necessary, experimental anaesthesia, euthanasia and disposal of these animals, year after year, can add up to a considerable sum. Many alternatives, on the other hand, can be used largely cost free, for years, once the initial purchase has been made. Often the initial sum required is not prohibitive. Most computer simulations, for example, are available for a few hundred dollars or less, and surgical or clinical task trainers can be considerably cheaper. The financial advantages of alternatives have been demonstrated in several studies (e.g., [15,16]), and are likely to become increasingly important as economic pressures on universities continue to rise in many countries.

Similar benefits have been demonstrated in terms of time savings. In his description of nerve physiology experiments, Clarke [17] provides some insights as to why:

"Previously, in such experiments, out of a typical allocated time of three hours, considerable time would be taken dissecting a viable sciatic nerve preparation and further time spent in trying to gain some small competence with the apparatus, at which point there would be a distinct possibility that the nerve was no longer viable (during the process of experimentation with the apparatus students often succeed in applying stimuli of enormous magnitude and frequency to the tissue). It is often a tired and irritable student who finally comes to the point in the experiment of measuring changes in response. Such a student is not in the optimum frame of mind to either perform the experiment with the due care and attention required or to think about the neurophysiological concepts involved. With the simulation, such problems are eliminated. Not only is much more time devoted to the experiment, but time is available to explore the subject in greater depth."

I can personally attest to the accuracy of the above comments, as this exact experiment was part of my veterinary physiology course when I was a student at Western Australia's Murdoch University in 1998. The experiences of my classmates were very similar to those described. Dissection of the nerves beforehand by technicians lessened, but did not eliminate, the considerable problems involved.

To further support this point, studies such as that by Dewhurst and Jenkinson [18] have demonstrated that computer simulations save teaching time, are less expensive, and can be effective and enjoyable mode of undergraduate biomedical student learning.

Overall, existing studies demonstrate time and cost benefits, rather than disadvantages, associated with humane alternatives (additional examples include [19,20]). Hence, complying with reasonable student requests for humane alternatives would be highly unlikely to incur financial or other burdens sufficient to jeopardise the continued operation of the institution—the necessary criterion for legally denying such a request on the basis of such burdens.

2.3. Claims of Educational Necessity

An educational institution such as a veterinary school might also attempt to deny a student's right to conscientiously object to certain animal use on the basis that such animal use is essential for educational purposes, and that without such use, the school would be unable to ensure the competency of the graduates produced. This is indeed valid with respect to some kinds of animal use, but not so with others. It is essential, for example, that veterinary students become competent at performing safe restraint, clinical examination and treatment of live animal patients. It is also essential that students gain sufficient knowledge of preclinical disciplines such as physiology, biochemistry and anatomy, as well as the practical skills required to provide surgical and medical interventions for patients. However, it does not necessarily follow that *harmful* animal use is required for the latter purposes.

A sizeable body of educational studies have compared the learning outcomes generated by non-harmful teaching methods with those achieved by harmful animal use. Of eleven studies of veterinary students published from 1989 to 2006 located during a recent survey [6], nine assessed surgical training. 45.5% (5/11) demonstrated superior learning outcomes using more humane alternatives. Another 45.5% (5/11) demonstrated equivalent learning outcomes, and 9.1% (1/11) demonstrated inferior learning outcomes. Twenty one studies of non-veterinary students in related academic disciplines were also published from 1968 to 2004. 38.1% (8/21) demonstrated superior, 52.4% (11/21) demonstrated equivalent, and 9.5% (2/21) demonstrated inferior learning outcomes using humane alternatives.

Twenty nine papers in which comparison with harmful animal use did not occur illustrated additional benefits of humane teaching methods in veterinary education, including: time and cost savings, enhanced potential for customisation and repeatability of the learning exercise, increased student confidence and satisfaction, increased compliance with animal use legislation, elimination of objections to the use of purpose-killed animals, and integration of clinical perspectives and ethics early in the curriculum [6].

These studies clearly indicate that if humane alternatives are well designed, they normally achieve learning outcomes as good, or in well over a third of all cases, better than those that rely on harmful animal use.

Additionally, there are numerous veterinary and other biomedical courses worldwide where alternatives are extensively and successfully used. Finally, explicit forms of animal use are not normally required by accreditation authorities. For example, the Australasian Veterinary Boards Council—which accredits veterinary schools in Australia and New Zealand—merely provides more general guidelines, such as "*Institutions need to demonstrate that students have supervised, intramural exposure to the major production and companion animal species relevant to veterinary professional activities in Australasia.*" [21]. As long as the educational institution produces graduates demonstrably competent in a set of specified skills and other competencies, institutions usually have considerable freedom about how they choose to teach them.

For these several reasons, any institution that attempted to deny a student's right to conscientiously object to harmful animal use on the basis of educational necessity would usually find itself in a weak position.

2.4. Adoption of Conscientious Objection Policies

Accordingly, veterinary schools and universities as a whole are increasingly acknowledging the validity of requests by students, and less often, faculty members, for humane teaching methods, and in several cases have established committees to examine these issues in depth. Policies allowing student conscientious objection, and formalising the process, have since been established at several veterinary schools.

The first formal, written policy adopted in an Australian veterinary school appears to have been that adopted by Western Australia's Murdoch University in 1998 (which has since been progressively updated; see Appendix), following a student campaign for humane teaching methods. The scope of this policy was not restricted to animal use, but covered any teaching or assessment activities to which students might conscientiously object, and was applicable to the university at large. Since then similar policies have been adopted at several other veterinary schools within Australia and abroad, such as those at the Universities of Sydney [22], Illinois at Urbana-Champaign [23], Queensland [24], and Adelaide [10], as well as by several other universities lacking veterinary faculties. In a majority of these examples conscientious objection policies are not restricted to the veterinary school, but are also applicable to other schools or programs, or to the university at large.

2.5. Definitions of Conscientious Objection

Should an institution choose to formulate a policy allowing student conscientious to certain forms of animal use, the definition of a conscientiously held belief will be one of its first, and most important, determinants. A definition that is too narrow in scope may prove insufficient to address legitimate student requests, prompting students to resort to the courts. One too broad may inadvertently allow a wider range of requests for alternate teaching and assessment activities than intended.

Fortunately, a body of legal precedent exists to inform such definitions. Australian courts have defined a conscientious belief as one based on a seriously and deeply held moral conviction, whether or not part of a religious doctrine or creed, and have stressed its durable, though not unchangeable, quality. The cases which have considered this issue have dealt primarily with conscientious objection to military service during the Vietnam War. Later cases adopting this definition have dealt with membership of Unions, and in a limited number of cases, with conscientious objection to jury service [25].

In two cases concerning conscientious objection to compulsory military service during the Vietnam War, the High Court of Australia approved a definition of conscientious objection previously provided by the Chief Justice of Western Australia [12]:

> *"Conscientious belief is an individual's inward conviction of what is morally right or morally wrong, and it is a conviction that is genuinely held after some process of thinking about the subject. It represents a conclusion that is uninfluenced by any consideration of*

personal advantage or disadvantage either to oneself or others, and perhaps when put to the test should be ordinarily combined with a willingness to act according to the particular conviction reached although this may involve personal discomfort or suffering or material loss."

2.6. 'Irrational' Beliefs

Those unfamiliar with this field often assume that a conscientiously held belief must be necessarily religious or rational. However, conscientious beliefs pertain to the moral convictions of individuals. Perhaps because the reasons and reasoning underpinning moral viewpoints varies so much between individuals, applicable case law has not generally required such beliefs to be rational in the eyes of other people.

For example, the NSW Law Reform Commission [12] has asserted that:

"In Australia various courts, tribunals and administrative officials have, over a substantial period, been required to test conscientious beliefs in the context of applications for exemption from civic duties imposed by legislation. The courts, in explaining this testing process, have been consistent in stating that the sole task of any person required to test a conscientious belief is to determine the genuineness of the particular applicant's conviction and not to consider the reasonableness, wisdom or correctness of its content."

Similarly, the Chief Justice of Tasmania, in an early compulsory national service case [12], stated:

"The only question I have to determine is whether the appellant does in fact conscientiously object to service ... And if I find that he does then my own view of the cogency or otherwise of the reasons upon which he holds the objection becomes immaterial, since it is of the essence of freedom of conscience that a man may hold to his conscientious conviction irrespective of whether a Judge or any other person thinks that he ought. Nor do I think that I should be too ready to impugn the bona fides of his objection because of some inconsistency in the views which he puts forward, or of evidence of instances of divergence between his behavior and his principles, since the compatibility of such phenomena with sincerity is unfortunately a commonplace of human experience."

This statement has been expressly approved by the Supreme Court of South Australia.

2.7. The Role of Religion

Similarly, although conscientiously held beliefs may indeed be religious, they are not required to be so to qualify as conscientiously held. This principle is not immediately obvious when examining some applicable legislation. Anti-discrimination (or 'equal opportunity') legislation, for example, often outlaws discrimination in the workplace or educational settings on the basis of political and religious beliefs. Discrimination on the basis of other beliefs is often not explicitly prohibited. The Western Australian Equal Opportunity Act (1984) [11] provides one such example.

However, as stated by the NSW Law Reform Commission Report [12],

"Some legislation has addressed religious objections exclusively. This reflects a view that a distinction can properly be drawn between a conscientious belief based on a religious doctrine and a conscientious belief not so based. However, the decided cases have affirmed that the term "conscience" of itself is not to be restricted by the ambit of "religion". Nor is the term "religion" to be defined restrictively. The Chief justice of the High Court of Australia warned in the Jehovah's Witness Case that "each person chooses the content of his own religion" and "[i]t is not for a court, upon some a priori basis, to disqualify certain beliefs as being incapable of being religious in character." (pp. 27–28).

This principle has been upheld by US courts, which wisely chose not to enter into the social debate about which beliefs qualify as religious—a debate the religious community itself has been unable to fully settle, despite hundreds of years of effort.

The NSW Law Reform Commission Report further states on p. 45 that,

"There appears to be no persuasive reason to restrict exemption to objectors on religious grounds. We consider that to do so would unjustifiably discriminate against those with sincere moral convictions which are unrelated to religious tenets."

This principle has been upheld in most Australian states when considering conscientious objection to jury service. Australia's Defence Legislation Amendment Act (1992) [26] states in Section 4 with respect to *"exemption from service because of conscientious beliefs… from combatant duties"*, that:

"a person is taken to have a conscientious belief in relation to a matter if the person's belief in respect of that matter:

(a) involves a fundamental conviction of what is morally right and morally wrong, whether or not based on religious considerations; and

(b) is so compelling in character for that person that he or she is duty bound to espouse it; and

(c) is likely to be of a long standing nature."

2.8. Definition of Conscientious Objection

Based on the jurisprudential principles previously described, a conscientiously held belief against participating in any nonessential teaching or assessment activity should comply with the following elements:

- Such a belief should represent be an individual's inward conviction of what is morally or religiously right or wrong.
- Such a belief need not qualify as rational in the eyes of others, or as a religious belief, although both may be true.
- Although when put to the test a conscientiously held belief should ordinarily be combined with a willingness to incur personal discomfort or suffering or material loss, the essence of non-discriminatory principles is that no student should be required to incur such losses, as a result of conscientiously objecting to participation in any nonessential educational activity. For the reasons provided previously, this clearly includes teaching or assessment activities involving harmful animal use.

3. Managing Conscientious Objection

Once agreement has been reached about which beliefs may be defined as conscientiously held, universities must decide how to assess conscientious objection claims, and what to do when a student request for alternate teaching and assessment activities is found to be based on conscientiously held belief. A range of approaches to these issues have been adopted by veterinary schools and universities.

3.1. Restrictive Approaches

A very few universities have chosen to adopt policies attempting to restrict enrolment to students that do not have conscientious objections to participating in harmful animal use within curricula. Examples include:

- Requiring students to sign an agreement on enrolment to the effect that they will participate in potentially objectionable activities, such as the dissection of purpose-killed animals, or experimentation on living animals.
- Requiring students to register their conscientious objection at time of application or enrolment.
- Screening students via their application forms and interviews in an attempt to exclude students who could conscientiously object to harmful animal use.

Adoption of such approaches potentially incurs several problems, however. First, if explicitly stated, such clearly discriminatory policies leave universities vulnerable to legal challenges. For example, as stated previously, in some circumstances the Western Australian Equal Opportunity Act (1984) [11] outlaws discrimination in education on the grounds of belief.

The publication of requirements that students must dissect purpose-killed animals, or experiment on living animals, also brings considerable potential for adverse publicity. The latter point is one universities are generally sensitive to, and was clearly illustrated in 2008 at Western Australia's Murdoch University. Within a short space of time Murdoch's attempt to require participation by two students in such harmful animal use resulted in significant adverse coverage for the university in both national television and national print media. Similar cases have occurred elsewhere.

Furthermore, students applying for admission to highly competitive courses such as veterinary science can be expected to be reluctant to admit any such concerns at the time of application or enrolment, reasonably fearing prejudicial treatment. An accurate picture could not be gained in this way.

Finally, one of the objectives of a university education is to teach students to think critically. It is a particular goal of most veterinary curricula to educate students about animal welfare issues, and to encourage students to think critically about these. Accordingly, it is hardly surprising that the beliefs of some students may evolve, and indeed change, over the duration of their veterinary courses, as they gain relevant knowledge and experience, and as their critical thinking skills progress.

Students initially supportive of harmful animal use within curricula may sometimes find themselves increasingly sceptical, and then opposed to such use. Such was the case at New Zealand's Massey University veterinary school when the opinions of third, fourth and fifth year veterinary students were surveyed in 2001, regarding the learning value of terminal physiology labs conducted in the third year of their veterinary curriculum [27]. In every one of nine questions about the educational value and ethical justification for these laboratory exercises, the attitudes of the fifth year students differed significantly from those of third year students. The authors concluded that, "*as the vet students are gaining experience their opinions appear to move systematically away from the position they held in year three.*" And, "*...the experiences of the vet students appear to be inducing doubt as to how justifiable is the use of live animals, relative to the knowledge and skill gained from the practise.*" Prior to this survey 68 sheep were killed annually. Partly due to these results, Massey University stated its intention to phase out these laboratories by 2004.

3.2. Inclusive Approaches

Other universities have formalized explicit policies welcoming students with a more diverse range of beliefs. Sometimes this is included within more general policies affirming equal educational opportunities for students from a diverse range of religious, cultural or other backgrounds. The discussion paper on student conscientious objection circulated at Murdoch University in 1998 provides a good example:

> "*The university is a public body whose mission includes a commitment to equity and to caring for its students*", and, "*By our very nature as a university, we are also committed to welcoming and respecting a range of ideas and beliefs, including those with which we may disagree.*" [25].

This ethos is reinforced by further statements within Murdoch's Handbook such as, "*Murdoch University is committed to equal opportunity and social justice principles, policy and practice through embedding social justice into academic business, maintaining an environment free from discrimination and supporting the diverse needs of students and staff.*" [28]. Murdoch has a dedicated website (http://our.murdoch.edu.au/Equal-opportunity-and-social-justice/) and a Student Equity and Social Justice Committee dedicated to realizing such ideals.

Such inclusive approaches have obvious benefits. They foster multiculturalism, increased understanding of, and tolerance for, differences, and may also yield public relations benefits in these respects. They are significantly more likely to comply with anti-discrimination legislation. They are more encouraging of the honest expression of student viewpoints on animal use issues, which in turn facilitates more honest discussion of these issues within animal welfare courses and elsewhere, creating better opportunities for student learning about animal welfare and animal ethics. And they avoid the potential for negative outcomes, including court challenges and adverse publicity, associated with more restrictive approaches.

3.3. Policy Recommendations

The *ad hoc* approach of many universities to conscientious objection frequently results in student requests for humane alternatives being made at late notice, increasing the likelihood such requests will be denied, and the chances of subsequent conflict; or alternatively, increases the likelihood that any alternatives provided will be suboptimal, due to insufficient preparation time. A formal policy and process pertaining to conscientious objection is therefore recommended, as it avoids such 'crisis management', and allows superior preparation and planning.

Social views on the acceptability of invasive curricular animal use are evolving, and it is predictable that student requests for humane alternatives are likely to increase, where such animal use remains. Accordingly, it is recommended that universities which include such curricular animal use should adopt and implement a formal policy allowing conscientious objection to educational activities that violate the conscientiously held beliefs of students. Alternative educational experiences and assessments should be provided for these students with the aim of providing equivalent outcomes in terms of knowledge and/or ability. These should require approximately equal commitments of time and effort, and in particular, should not be punitively burdensome, with the capacity to demonstrate this in case of scrutiny or challenge.

Although universities should generally accommodate requests for alternate teaching or assessment activities where participation would require a student to violate a conscientiously held belief (such as against unnecessarily harming animals), this does not mean that all requests should be accommodated. In particular, universities should not accommodate requests if by doing so they would violate a law (e.g., demands for racial segregation due to beliefs based on racism).

Finally, in the event that a student's request is denied or the student is unsatisfied with the alternative offered, an appeals process should be available.

3.4. Publication of Policies

Well prior to the commencement of any course in which animals are used, information about animal use and the university policies pertaining to conscientious objection should be published in writing to all students taking applicable courses. This information should be provided within student handbooks, curricular and course guides, and any other appropriate information outlets.

The university handbook should include a section on conscientious objection, which details the conscientious objection policy, provides the university definition of a conscientiously held belief, describes the procedure for registering a conscientious objection to participating in a teaching or assessment activity, and the procedure for assessing claims of conscientious objection, and details the appeals process.

Students should be advised to seek information as early as possible about educational activities to which they might have a conscientious objection, from any applicable curricular guides, and particularly, any course descriptions or materials such as laboratory descriptions, as well as from the student handbook, Course Coordinators, or their Program Chairs or Heads of School. Students should be advised of the benefits of early notification; particularly, that this will allow sufficient time for their claims to be assessed, and for alternatives to be sourced and prepared, and will decrease the likelihood that suboptimal activities will be provided. Students should be requested to raise their claims of conscientious objection with their Course Coordinators, Program Chairs or Heads of School as early as possible, and preferably before the start of semester, although this will be determined to some extent by the date of release of course materials describing curricular animal use and conscientious objection policies.

To facilitate this process, course and curricular materials should aim to summarise information on potentially objectionable activities occurring within any courses. In the case of animal usage, this information should include all of the following:

- which courses animals are used in
- what species and numbers of animals are used
- how the animals are sourced
- a summary of the procedures carried out on them (e.g., dissection, experimentation on living animals or organs sourced from them, non-recovery surgery)
- why the animals are considered necessary
- details of any refinement methods used (to decrease suffering, and maximise well-being, such as analgesics or environmental enrichment)
- details of their housing or caging on or off campus, prior to and after use
- whether and how the animals are euthanized and disposed of

All of this information may be necessary to allow students to properly consider whether or not they conscientiously object to activities involving these animals.

A minority of poorly prepared students may only become aware of the depth of their objection to an activity when physically confronted with it (e.g., in the case of highly invasive experiments on living animals), and the university may still be obliged to cater for them. Therefore, there the absolute cut-off date for raising claims of conscientious objection should be the date of the objectionable activity in question. It is not reasonable for any student to request an alternative to an activity in which they've already chosen to participate, on the basis that they conscientiously objected to it. It is important to bear in mind that this defence may not apply, however, if a student is able to reasonably claim they were coerced into participating, by the application of any undue pressure by faculty, for example. However, it should be made quite clear that the quality of alternatives provided to students may well depend on the amount of time they give staff to prepare them. Staff should also be directed to consider in advance what alternatives they might provide, should students raise objections to participating in activities within their courses.

3.5. Assessing Claims of Conscientious Objection

Claims of conscientious objection should be initially assessed by the Course Coordinator, or, where the issue is systemic to the units offered within a programme, by an appropriate official such as the Programme Chair or Head of School.

Students voicing a conscientious objection should normally be initially required to meet with the appropriate official concerned, who should seek to clarify what activity the student is seeking to object to, exactly which aspects of the procedure they are objecting to (e.g., the species used? the invasiveness of the procedure? the killing of an animal?), and whether any mitigating factors might be sufficient to overcome these objections, such as the use of a species of lower sentience, a less invasive procedure, or the use of analgesics or anesthetics. The latter information might be important in seeking to establish an acceptable alternative teaching or assessment activity. To determine whether the objection(s) are truly conscientiously held, or merely elicit feelings of discomfort, for example, the official should also seek to determine the depth of the student's convictions, by careful questioning. As stated previously, an acceptable definition of a conscientiously held belief is that when put to the test such a belief should ordinarily be combined with a willingness to incur personal discomfort, suffering or material loss. However, the essence of non-discriminatory principles is that no student should be required to incur such losses, as a result of their conscientiously objection.

To increase the transparency and defensibility of these proceedings, it is also advisable to ensure at least one additional faculty member or university official is present as a witness. The student should also be offered the opportunity to invite a friend, colleague or family member in support.

At the beginning of the meeting, the process for assessing claims of conscientious objection, and in particular the type of questions to be asked and the need to ask them, should be explained to all parties, who should also be reminded of the university's commitment to maintaining the confidentiality of personal information pertaining to students. In the interest of maintaining written case records, at the end of the meeting students should perhaps be asked to follow up with a written description of their conscientious objection and a formal request for alternatives. At the end of this process of assessment a decision should be made about what alternatives will be offered to accommodate the student's request, or to instead deny the request.

Students whose claims are denied or who are dissatisfied with these assessments and educational experiences subsequently offered should have access to an avenue of appeal. Given the potential legal implications for the university where conscientious objectors are discriminated against, appeals committees should include a lawyer, ideally with relevant expertise, possibly from the university's law faculty, if such exists.

3.6. Related Considerations

Faculty members assessing claims of conscientious objection should be appraised of the details of the university's conscientious objection policy, including the agreed definition of conscientiously held beliefs, the procedure for assessing claims of conscientious objection, and of the appeals process. In particular such faculty should be reminded that conscientious beliefs need not have a religious or rational basis, and of the desirability of showing respect to all beliefs, including those with which they might personally disagree. Their sole objectives should be to determine whether or not the beliefs in question are conscientiously held, and if so, what alternatives to the objectionable activities can be provided, given concurrent requirements to ensure the curriculum continues to meet any applicable accreditation standards. Faculty should understand that they must not seek to cross examine students unduly, nor seek to alter their beliefs.

Finally, records should be kept of all cases of student conscientious objection, sufficient to support a defence in the event of legal challenge, as well as to support educational studies, such as those examining student learning outcomes using different teaching methodologies. These should include, at a minimum, details such as the nature of the conscientiously held belief(s), the activities objected to, alternatives provided, educational performance of the student at that time, at the end of the course, and within the degree overall as assessed at the time of graduation, as well as the dates of all relevant events, and the names of all involved.

4. Conclusions

The right of an individual to act in accordance with their conscience or belief is often considered fundamentally important within modern democracies, with the result that it may legally be violated only in the gravest of circumstances, such as national emergencies. With respect to student (or, less commonly, faculty) beliefs against participating in activities involving animals, it is likely that a university could legally require such conscientious objectors to violate their beliefs on penalty of academic sanction, only if it could demonstrate to the satisfaction of a court that participation in such activities was truly necessary to ensure the competency of the graduates produced, or alternatively, that accommodating such beliefs would incur financial or administrative burdens so severe as so seriously threaten the continued operation of the institution. However, when alternatives are requested to harmful animal use, a considerable body of existing evidence suggests financial and time-related benefits, rather than disadvantages, associated with humane teaching methods. Because of such factors, it highly unlikely such a case could be won in a court of law.

Additionally, because of changing knowledge pertaining to the sentience and other psychosocial characteristics relevant to the moral status of animals, as well as changing social attitudes toward animals and changing student demographics, and the on-going development of humane teaching methods, conscientious objection to harmful animal use within veterinary and other biomedical faculty are likely to continue to increase over time.

Accordingly, it is recommended that those universities offering relevant courses that have not yet done so, proceed to implement policies agreeing to make reasonable accommodations for students (or staff) who conscientiously object to participating in harmful animal use.

Formalisation of such policies has several advantages. Such formal policies demonstrate institutional commitment to fostering a culture which is tolerant of diversity, and respects a range of viewpoints, beliefs and backgrounds. They can increase compliance with applicable legislation outlawing certain forms of discrimination in education or the workplace. They greatly decrease the likelihood of conflicts relating to curricular animal use, which can be extremely damaging to the careers of the students or others involved, and to the reputation of the university at large. And they maximise the likelihood of honest disclosure of student concerns, and of prior warning of incidents, and minimise crisis management or *ad hoc* responses.

Once adopted, detailed information about curricular animal use and related conscientious objection policies, including the appeals process, should be publicised to all students via university handbooks, curricular and course guides, and any other appropriate information outlets, well prior to the commencement of courses in which animals are used. Such information should also be circulated to faculty, along with guidelines about assessing conscientious objection claims, and the provision of alternative teaching or assessment activities. Faculty should be reminded that applicable case law does not require conscientiously held beliefs to be rational or religious in the eyes of other people, and of the wisdom and necessity of not exerting undue pressure on such students, and of showing respect for beliefs with which they may personally disagree.

Conflicts of Interest

The author declares no conflict of interest.

References

1.   Rowan, A.N. The use of alternatives in veterinary training. In *Animals in Biomedical Research. Replacement, Reduction and Refinement: Present Possibilities and Future Prospects*; Hendriksen, F.M., Koeter, H.B.W.M., Eds.; Elsevier Science Publishers: Amsterdam, The Netherlands, 1991; pp. 127–139.

2.   Bauer, M.S. A survey of the use of live animals, cadavers, inanimate models, and computers in teaching veterinary surgery. *J. Amer. Vet. Med. Assoc.* **1993**, *203*, 1047–1051.

3.   Knight, A. Alternatives to harmful animal use in tertiary education. *Altern. Lab. Anim.* **1999**, *27*, 967–974.

4.   Gruber, F.P.; Dewhurst, D.G. Alternatives to animal experimentation in biomedical education. *ALTEX* **2004**, *21(Suppl. 1)*, 33–48.

5.   Martinsen, S.; Jukes, N. Towards a humane veterinary education. *J. Vet. Med. Educ.* **2006**, *32*, 454–460.

6.   Knight, A. The effectiveness of humane teaching methods in veterinary education. *ALTEX* **2007**, *24*, 91–109.

7.   Romano, M. CU settles suit over dog experiments. *Rocky Mountain News* 1 September 1995.

8.   Balcombe, J. Student/teacher conflict regarding animal dissection. *Amer. Biol. Teach.* **1997**, *59*, 22–25.

9.   Francione, G.; Charlton, A. *Vivisection and Dissection in the Classroom: A Guide to Conscientious Objection*; American Anti-Vivisection Society: Philadelphia, PA, USA, 1992.

10. Whittaker, A.; Anderson, G. A policy at the University of Adelaide for student objections to the use of animals in teaching. *J. Vet. Med. Educ.* **2013**, *40*, 52–57.

11. The Equal Opportunity Commission of Western Australia. The Equal Opportunity Act 1984, Section 61. Perth, Australia, 2010. Available online: http://www.eoc.wa.gov.au/AboutUs/ TheEqualOpportuntiyAct.aspx (accessed on 18 December 2013).

12. New South Wales Law Reform Commission. *Community Law Reform Programme. Sixth Report: Conscientious Objection to Jury Service*; New South Wales Law Reform Commission: Sydney, Australia, 1984.

13. Centre for Human Rights. *The International Bill of Human Rights*; United Nations: Geneva, Switzerland, 1996; p. 25.

14. Balcombe, J. A global overview of law and policy concerning animal use in education. In *Progress in the Reduction, Refinement and Replacement of Animal Experimentation*; Balls, M., Zeller, A.-M., Halder, M.E., Eds.; Elsevier: New York, NY, USA, 2000; pp. 1343–1350.

15. Henman, C.; Leach, G. An alternative method for pharmacology laboratory class instruction using Biovideograph video tape recordings. *Brit. J. Pharmacol.* **1983**, *80*, 591P.

16. Dewhurst, D.; Hardcastle, J.; Hardcastle, P.; Stuart, E. Comparison of a computer simulation program and a traditional laboratory practical class for teaching the principles of intestinal absorption. *Amer. J. Physiol.* **1994**, *267*, S95–S104.

17. Clarke, K. The use of microcomputer simulations in undergraduate neurophysiology experiments. *Altern. Lab. Anim.* **1987**, *14*, 134–140.

18. Dewhurst, D.; Jenkinson, L. The impact of computer-based alternatives on the use of animals in undergraduate teaching. *Altern. Lab. Anim.* **1995**, *23*, 521–530.

19. Rudas, P. Hypermedia in veterinary education. In *Proceedings of the 3rd Annual International Conference and Exhibition on CAD/CAM/CAE/CIM. Applications for Manufacturing and Productivity*; Hencsey, G., Renner, G., Eds.; World Computer Graphics Association: Budapest, Hungary, 1993; pp. 212–218.

20. Dhein, C.R.; Memon, M. On-line continuing education at the College of Veterinary Medicine, Washington State University. *J. Vet. Med. Educ.* **2003**, *30*, 41–46.

21. Australasian Veterinary Boards Council Inc (AVBC). *AVBC—Policies, Procedures & Standards*; AVBC: Melbourne, Australia, 2010.

22. McGreevy, P.D.; Dixon, R.J. Teaching animal welfare at the University of Sydney's Faculty of Veterinary Science. *J. Vet. Med. Educ.* **2005**, *32*, 442–446.

23. Knight, A. Humane teaching methods in veterinary education. *Aust. Vet. J.* **2007**, *85*, N28–N29.

24. University of Queensland School of Veterinary Science. *University of Queensland School of Veterinary Science Guidelines on Ethical Concerns on Use of Animals in Teaching*; University of Queensland School of Veterinary Science: Gatton, Queensland, Australia, 2008. Available online: http://www.humanelearning.info/resources/conscientious_objection.htm (accessed on 3 November 2013).

25. Murdoch University. *Conscientious Objection in Teaching and Assessment: Report of the Working Party*; Murdoch University: Perth, Australia, 1998.

26. Australian Government. *Defence. Legislation Amendment Act.* (1992). Available online: http://www.comlaw.gov.au/Details/C2004A04382 (accessed on 19 December 2013).

27. Massey University. *2001 Veterinary Student Report*; Massey University: Palmerston North, New Zealand, 2001. Available online: http://www.humanelearning.info/resources/surveys.htm (accessed on 3 November 2013).

28. Murdoch University. *Handbook 2013*; Murdoch University: Perth, Australia, 2013. Available online: http://handbook.murdoch.edu.au/_files/authoritative_handbook_2013.pdf (accessed on 3 November 2013).

29. Murdoch University. *Conscientious Objection in Teaching and Assessment Policy*; Murdoch University: Perth, Australia, 2012. Available online: https://policy.murdoch.edu.au/ Default.aspx?auto=false&public=true (accessed on 3 November 2013).

Appendix

Conscientious Objection in Teaching and Assessment Policy
Murdoch University, Western Australia

Initially approved 11 November 1998
Current version approved 8 August 2012 [29]

Purpose

To provide guidance to students and staff dealing with situations where conscientious belief conflicts with unit requirements.

Policy

1. The University recognises that some students may have a conscientious belief which is in conflict with learning activities, including those for assessment, in one or more units in which they enrol. The University shall endeavour to make reasonable accommodations to meet such beliefs. Notwithstanding the provisions of this policy, the University will not act in any way that violates Commonwealth or State law and the University is not obliged to accommodate a conscientious belief which puts it at risk of violating a law (e.g., a belief based on racism).

2. In considering such cases, the University accepts that conscientious belief is a genuine and sustained conviction of what may be morally right or wrong that is uninfluenced by any consideration of personal advantage or disadvantage to either the student themselves or others in pursuit of their course of study. This conviction can be based on religious reasons, belief in the sanctity of life, environmental concerns, or other reasons that the student deems central to their belief system.

3. The onus is on the student to take the initiative in identifying a conscientious difficulty with a learning activity, including those for assessment and to draw this to the attention of the University before undertaking such practice. [A student cannot appeal against a practice which he or she has already undertaken.] It is preferable for students with a conscientious objection to be identified early, so there is time to assess it and to make any necessary arrangements. Wherever possible, students with a conscientious objection in a unit should raise their difficulties with the Unit Coordinator prior to the start of the unit or in the first three weeks of semester. If the difficulty is with units in future semesters or is systemic to units offered in the course, the student should discuss this with the Academic Chair as early as possible. It is for these staff to assess whether the claim constitutes a conscientious objection and what arrangements can be made to accommodate it. The staff member has the discretion to ask for more information from the student in order to establish whether or not the student has a conscientious belief.

4. In cases where Unit Coordinators can foresee students having problems of belief in their unit, the unit study guide should mention these and advise any students with problems about this to see the Unit Coordinator.

5. The student can request that there be a suitable alternative, but has no right to demand that the alternative take a particular form. There are also countervailing factors to be taken into account in deciding whether and (if so) how to meet the student's concerns, including:

   - professional requirements: those of external registration bodies, and staff concerns to be able to certify that graduates have met the course learning outcomes and basic professional competencies. This requires a careful consideration of whether or not the learning activity or assessment at issue is essential for the training of practitioners in that profession.

- whether it is a required or an elective unit (the case for expensive alternative arrangements in an elective unit is much weaker)
- whether there is time to put alternative arrangements in place
- whether it would result in the University breaching its equal opportunity obligations
- whether other students would be disadvantaged in the quality of their education
- cost.

6. Students with a conscientious objection to a particular learning activity, including those for assessment, should not simply be excused from an activity, but instead be given an alternative that meets the same learning outcomes. Alternatives made available to students with a conscientious objection do not have to be made available to all other students in the unit.

7. A Unit Coordinator who has considered and approved a student case of conscientious objection must advise the Enrolments and Fees of this, giving details of the nature of the conscientious belief and the alternative arrangements made for loading into the student record system.

8. Unit Coordinators should ensure that the alternative arrangements made for similar conscientious objections are consistent.

9. A student who is dissatisfied with the decision of the Unit Coordinator may request the School Dean to review the decision and thereafter appeal to the Student Appeals Committee.

7

A Critical Look at Biomedical Journals' Policies on Animal Research by Use of a Novel Tool: The EXEMPLAR Scale

Ana Raquel Martins [1] and Nuno Henrique Franco [2,*]

[1] Faculty of Sciences, University of Porto, Rua do Campo Alegre S/N, 4169-007 Porto, Portugal;
E-Mail: up201101588@fc.up.pt

[2] IBMC—Instituto de Biologia Molecular e Celular, University of Porto, Rua do Campo Alegre 823, 4150-180 Porto, Portugal

* Author to whom correspondence should be addressed; E-Mail: nfranco@ibmc.up.pt

Academic Editor: Clive J. C. Phillips

Simple Summary: Biomedical journals have the responsibility to promote humane research. To gauge and evaluate journal policies on animal research, the *EXEMPLAR*—For "Excellence in Mandatory Policies on Animal Research"—scale is presented and applied to evaluate a sample of 170 biomedical journals, providing an overview of the current landscape of editorial policies on the ethical treatment of animals.

Abstract: Animal research is not only regulated by legislation but also by self-regulatory mechanisms within the scientific community, which include biomedical journals' policies on animal use. For editorial policies to meaningfully impact attitudes and practice, they must not only be put into effect by editors and reviewers, but also be set to high standards. We present a novel tool to classify journals' policies on animal use—the *EXEMPLAR* scale—as well as an analysis by this scale of 170 journals publishing studies on animal models of three human diseases: Amyotrophic Lateral Sclerosis, Type-1 Diabetes and Tuberculosis. Results show a much greater focus of editorial policies on regulatory compliance than on other domains, suggesting a transfer of journals' responsibilities to scientists, institutions and regulators. Scores were not found to vary with journals' impact factor, country of origin or antiquity, but were, however, significantly higher for open access journals, which may be a result of their greater exposure and consequent higher public scrutiny.

Keywords: animal research; animal ethics; animal welfare; editorial policies; EXEMPLAR scale

1. Introduction

Animal experimentation has, for centuries, not only been a cornerstone of scientifically-based biomedical research, but also the subject of heated academic and public debate [1]. Given the number and complexity of the arguments at play in this discussion, views on the moral acceptability of animal experiments are diverse, most of which fall in between the diametrically opposed views of those uncompromisingly against this practice and the more determined advocates of animal experimentation. Such diversity results from the interplay between such factors—among others—as the suffering and discomfort endured by animals [2–4], the purpose and validity of research [4–8], which species are used [6,9–11] or the degree of confidence in scientists and regulators [3,12,13], as well as the different positions on the weighting that should be given to each factor.

In spite of this multitude of positions, in western societies, the majority of the public tends to follow a moderate, mainstream view on the subject, according to which animal experimentation is seen as a legitimate and ethically acceptable scientific activity, provided it is guided by a scientifically sound and medically relevant objective, and that animal welfare is taken into consideration [8,13]. This "conditional approval" view is in line with the tenet of the Three Rs [14]—for the Replacement, Reduction and Refinement of animal use in science—widely accepted as a scientifically sound approach to help address the ethical dilemma put forth by animal research [8,15], as well as an overarching principle in current European legislation regulating animal use for scientific purposes [16].

The mandate of scientists to work with animals requires a continually renewed relationship of trust with society, whose views and expectations, on the other hand, legislators also take into account when establishing the legal framework within which scientists must work. This tacit "social license" granted to scientists warrants public trust in the relevance, competency, reliability, ethicality and transparency of animal experiments, which goes beyond the mere assumption of compliance with laws and regulations [17,18]. From this interplay results a tightly regulated environment for animal research, by both 'external' regulatory frameworks (such as legislation [16,19]) and self-regulatory initiatives from within the scientific community itself. These include peer review [20], training [21,22], the issuing of publication guidelines (such as ARRIVE [23] or the *Gold Standard Publication Checklist* [24]) or other scientific community-driven initiatives, such as the Basel Declaration for transparency in animal research [25]. Biomedical journals' policies also have great potential for improving principles and practice in animal research, since the motivation—and often the pressure—to publish may serve as an incentive for scientists to comply with journals' demands [26,27] on such issues as quality of research and reporting, or the ethical treatment of animals, particularly for high-impact journals.

Given the potential of scientific journals for promoting best practice in animal research, evaluating their level of concern for animal welfare and the quality of research becomes of the essence. In 2009, RSPCA's Nicola Osborne *et al.* [28] proposed a 12-item (each awarding one point) classifying scheme for scoring biomedical journals' policies on animal welfare and the Three Rs, and presented results of a review of 236 biomedical journals' policies. They found that in 35% of their sample, animal use was not even contemplated in the guidelines for authors or anywhere else, in 18% animals were mentioned in some way but no perceptible guidelines were provided and the remaining scored rather poorly, with 37% scoring three or fewer points (out of 12).

Table 1. The Excellence in Editorial Mandatory Policies for Animal Research (EXEMPLAR) scale.

EXEMPLAR Scale		Score
A—Reporting of regulatory compliance		
Authors must attest of prior ethical approval of animal studies, or an analogous project evaluation process involving harm-benefit appraisal, (e.g., by providing documental evidence or ethics review board process reference) and include a statement of compliance with relevant legislation and national, international or institutional guidelines on animal care and use.		**5**
Authors must declare:	Ethical approval of studies or analogous evaluation process by competent authority, institutional animal care and use committee, animal welfare body or equivalent.	2
	Compliance with relevant national, international or institutional guidelines on animal care and use.	1
	Compliance with relevant legislation on the use of animals.	1
B—Quality of research and reporting of results		
Journal refers authors to relevant guidelines on the quality of reporting of animal studies (e.g., ARRIVE guidelines, Gold Standard Publication Checklist, or other)		**5**
Authors must include information regarding:	Animals (e.g., sex, age, genotype, background, supplier, acclimatization period, *etc.*)	1
	Experimental conditions (e.g., housing, lighting, temperature, feeding regime, environmental enrichment, *etc.*)	1
	Experimental design and statistics	1
	Experimental procedures and outcomes	1
C—Animal Welfare and ethics		
Journal demands that the methods described are coherent with best principles and practice on the ethical treatment of animals in research, e.g., by demanding strict compliance with relevant guidelines on animal care and use, the 3Rs for *replacement*, *reduction* and *refinement* or the journal's own policies.		**5**
Authors must:	state the rationale for choosing the animal model(s) used	1
	report the impact of the experiment on animal health and wellbeing	1
	describe any measures to minimize harm (e.g., anesthetics, analgesics, humane endpoints) and/or improve the wellbeing of animals (e.g., husbandry adaptations for more vulnerable animals)	1
	justify the necessity of any unrelieved pain, suffering or distress inflicted	1
D—Criteria for the exclusion of papers		
Meeting journal standards on animal ethics care and welfare is indispensable for manuscript acceptance and/or publication. Studies raising serious concerns over animal welfare, or presenting significant discrepancies between the approved protocol and methods described may be reported to the institution or committee responsible for ethical approval.		**5**
Studies raising serious ethical concerns (e.g., serious neglect regarding animal welfare or unjustifiable suffering considering the value of the experiment) may be rejected by editors or reviewers.		3
Journal states specific procedure(s) that will not be accepted for publication (e.g., use of muscle relaxants or paralytic drugs alone for surgery, severe lesion/trauma without anesthesia, or death as an endpoint)		1

The present study presents the "EXEMPLAR"—an acronym for "Excellence in Editorial Mandatory Policies for Animal Research"—Scale (Table 1) as a novel approach and tool to classify and evaluate scientific journals' editorial policies on animal use. The EXEMPLAR Scale aims to (a) gauge the consideration (or lack thereof) given by journals to the most relevant aspects of animal use in the life sciences; (b) present a novel way for scoring editorial policies and (c) propose a set of ideal standards for three key aspects in which journal policies can have an instrumental role in promoting best practice: regulatory compliance, quality of reporting and animal welfare and ethics; along with a fourth category for the enforcement of said policies.

This paper also presents an overview of the current landscape of biomedical journals' policies, by reviewing and classifying by the EXEMPLAR a sample of 170 journals publishing animal studies within three fields of biomedical research: Amyotrophic Lateral Sclerosis (ALS), Type 1 Diabetes (T1D) and Tuberculosis (TB). These fields were selected for being the subject of ongoing systematic reviews in our lab—which will later allow for a comparison between the principles reflected in explicit policies and the actual practice patent in the articles published by the journals in our sample—which in turn were selected for representing areas in which animal experimentation is recurrent and widespread.

2. Experimental Section

2.1. The Exemplar Scale

The EXEMPLAR scale (Table 1) was developed to classify scientific journals' editorial policies on animal studies, scoring them from zero to 20 points. The scale is divided into four categories, each of them regarding a relevant aspect of journal policies on animal research. The maximum score for each category is five points, granted to journals that uphold to the scale's gold-standard for that category. For any journal not abiding to the category's "gold-standard" criterion, up to four points can be attributed if it nevertheless abides to other relevant criteria listed for that category, each deemed a "standard" criterion.

Categories are divided as such: Category A—Regulatory compliance; Category B—Quality of research and reporting of results, Category C—Animal welfare and ethics; Category D—Criteria for exclusion of papers. Both Categories B and C have four standard criteria, each one worth one point. Category A has three standard criteria, with the item "authors must declare ethical approval of studies or analogous project evaluation process (…)" awarding two points. This is based on the assumptions that (a) project approval involves some level of harm-benefit appraisal by a third party—such as the competent authority or an ethics committee—and (b) that the latter is of greater significance for the humane treatment of animals than plain self-reported compliance with laws and legislation. Category D only has two standard criteria, one of which awarding three points to journals which state that papers may be reject upon ethical concerns. This also follows the rationale that some criteria are of greater relevance than others, in this case, the mere listing of procedures the journal is not willing to publish.

For reporting purposes, the overall EXEMPLAR score is presented along with a breakdown of the partial scores for each category, allowing for anyone knowledgeable of the scale to identify in which dimensions a given journal's policy is stronger or, on the other hand, where further development is due. For example, the hypothetical *EXEMPLAR score = 12: (A-5; B-5; C-2; D-0)*—or *12:(5,5,2,0)*—would suggest that the journal in question follows "gold standard" criteria for both Categories A and B, that it fulfils half the criteria for Category C and that no policies regarding Category D are described.

2.2. Journals Search

A list of papers reporting studies on murine models of Type-1 Diabetes (T1D), Tuberculosis (TB) and Amyotrophic Lateral Sclerosis (ALS) published between 2011 and 2013 was retrieved by a ISI Web of Science™ (Core Collection v5.13.1) advanced search. The search was carried out in April 2014 using the queries *TS= (("NOD mouse" OR "NOD mice" OR "non obese diabetic" OR "nonobese diabetic") AND diabet*)*; *TS = ((mice OR mouse) AND tuberculosis)*; and *TS = ((mice OR mouse) SAME (ALS OR "amyotrophic lateral sclerosis"))*. The results were refined to only include articles in English reporting original research, and afterwards downloaded and archived as an ENDNOTE® database. After being refined, search results were as such: T1D: 655 papers; TB: 1107 papers; ALS: 1114 papers. The criterion for selecting which journals to classify was to only include those that had published three or more papers in each field over the time period selected (Figure 1). This resulted in a sample of 44 journals for T1D (which published 475/655, or 73%, of T1D papers retrieved); 65 journals for TB (which published 999/1107, or 72% of all TB papers retrieved) and 84 journals for ALS (which published 830/1114, or 75%, of all ALS papers retrieved).

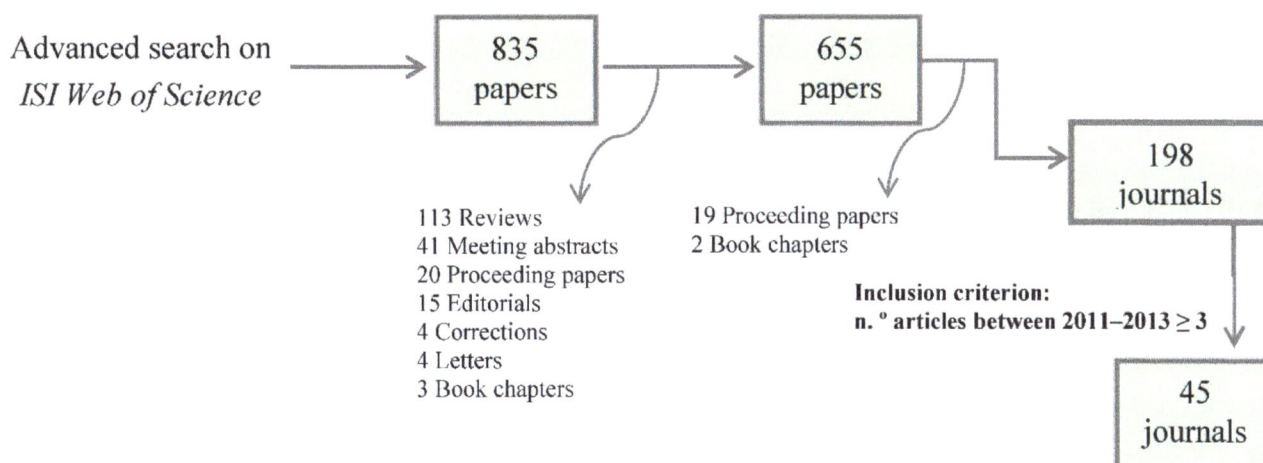

Figure 1. Schematic representation of the search and selection process, with the search for journals publishing studies on Type 1 Diabetes (T1D) being presented as an example. One of the journals from the T1D sample was later excluded because their editorial polices stated that it did not publish studies on animal models, leaving a final sample size of 44 journals.

2.3. Data Collection

Journal policies were collected by finding the "authors guidelines", "Instructions for authors" sections or equivalent on each journal's website, and saving them to a database. Whenever a journal required authors to comply with general policies of its publishing house, or subscribed to other guidelines (e.g., by the International Association of Veterinary Editors), these were also considered as a part of the journal's policies.

General information on each journal—impact factor, publisher, country and scientific category—were collected from the ISI Web of Knowledge Journal Citation Reports®, JCR Science Edition 2013, while information regarding the date (year) of the first issue and model of publication—*i.e.*, subscription based *vs.* open access—were retrieved from each journal's website. Only journals in which all published papers were readily and freely accessible without any embargo period were considered to be "open access".

All editorial policies were classified according to both the EXEMPLAR Scale (Table 1) and the classification scheme proposed by Osborne *et al.* [28].

2.4. Statistical Analysis

Chi-square tests were conducted to assess the relationship between the EXEMPLAR Score (ES) and qualitative variables (model of publication, country, and publisher), while for quantitative variables (impact factor, first year of edition and the score by the Osborne *et al.* scale) a logistic regression analysis was also performed. Linear relationships were assessed by the Pearson test. For some non-parametric statistical tests, the variable "ES" was transformed into a dichotomous variable, ES < eight and ES ≥ eight. A score of eight points was selected as a threshold for a minimally acceptable policy on animal use, since it can be awarded to a journal that complies with half the "standard" criteria defined for each category. Statistical analysis was conducted using SPSS Statistics 22 (IBM, Armonk, NY, USA; version 22.0).

3. Results and Discussion

3.1. Sample Characterization

The total sample comprised 170 journals, published by 54 academic publishers, with headquarters in 20 countries. Four publishers were responsible for publishing nearly half (49%) of the retrieved journals, namely Elsevier (36 journals), Wiley-Blackwell (22 journals), Springer (13 journals) and Nature Publishing Group (12 journals). Regarding country of origin, 95% of all journals were either based in the EU (81/170, 47 of which in the United Kingdom and 11 in the Netherlands) or the United States of America (USA) (80/170). The mean impact factor of the journals in this sample was 4.79 (Median = 3.63; Standard Deviation = 3.85). The median year of publication of first issue was 1987, with 75% of journals preceding 2002. Figure 2 represents the distribution of journals by field of research (of the three fields reviewed for this present study).

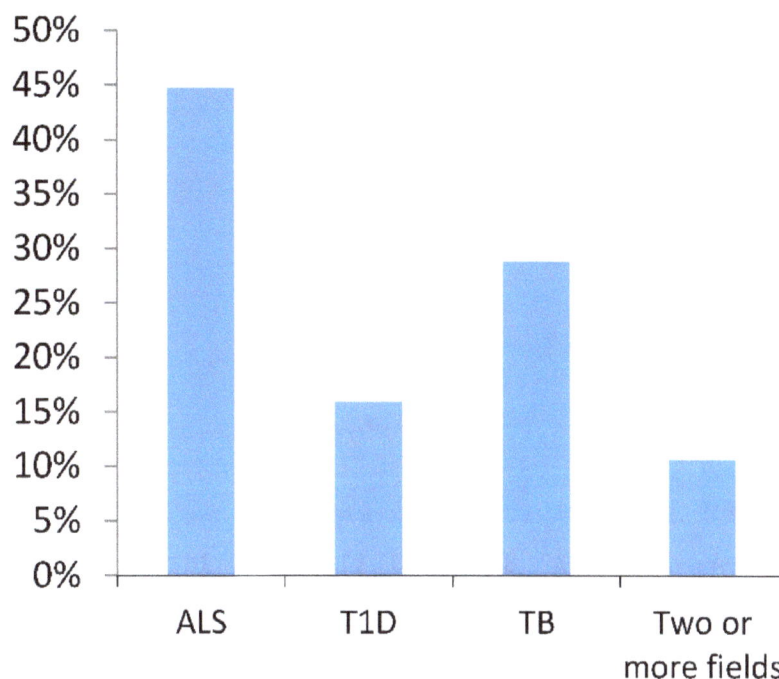

Figure 2. Topics covered by the journals in the sample (of the three selected). Journals publishing studies in more than one of the selected fields (n = 18) included two journals publishing papers on T1D and ALS, one journal publishing on Amyotrophic Lateral Sclerosis (ALS) and Tuberculosis (TB), ten journals publishing on both T1D and TB and five journals publishing papers on all three fields, between 2011–2013.

3.2. EXEMPLAR Score

No significant differences were found between the scores of the three sub-samples analyzed, the same happening for score distribution (Figure 3B). Results are hence presented for all journals pooled ($N = 170$, after removing duplicate entries from journals publishing in more than one field), unless stated otherwise. Category A ("reporting of regulatory compliance") registered the highest non-nil score of all categories (92%), with 5% of journals being awarded the top score of five points. As for Category B ("Quality of research and reporting of results"), 72% had a nil score. However, 18% of journals were awarded the top score for this category, virtually all of these for referring to the ARRIVE guidelines. As for Category C (Ethical treatment of animals) and Category D (Criteria for the exclusion of papers), 86% and 91% of journals scored zero points, respectively (Figure 4). Overall, only 18% (31/170) of journals scored eight points or higher, with the two top-scoring journals being published by the Public Library of Science (*PLOS*), namely *PLOS One*, with a maximum score of 20 points, and *PLOS Genetics*, which scored 15 points (the two other PLOS journals in the sample scored five and 10 points).

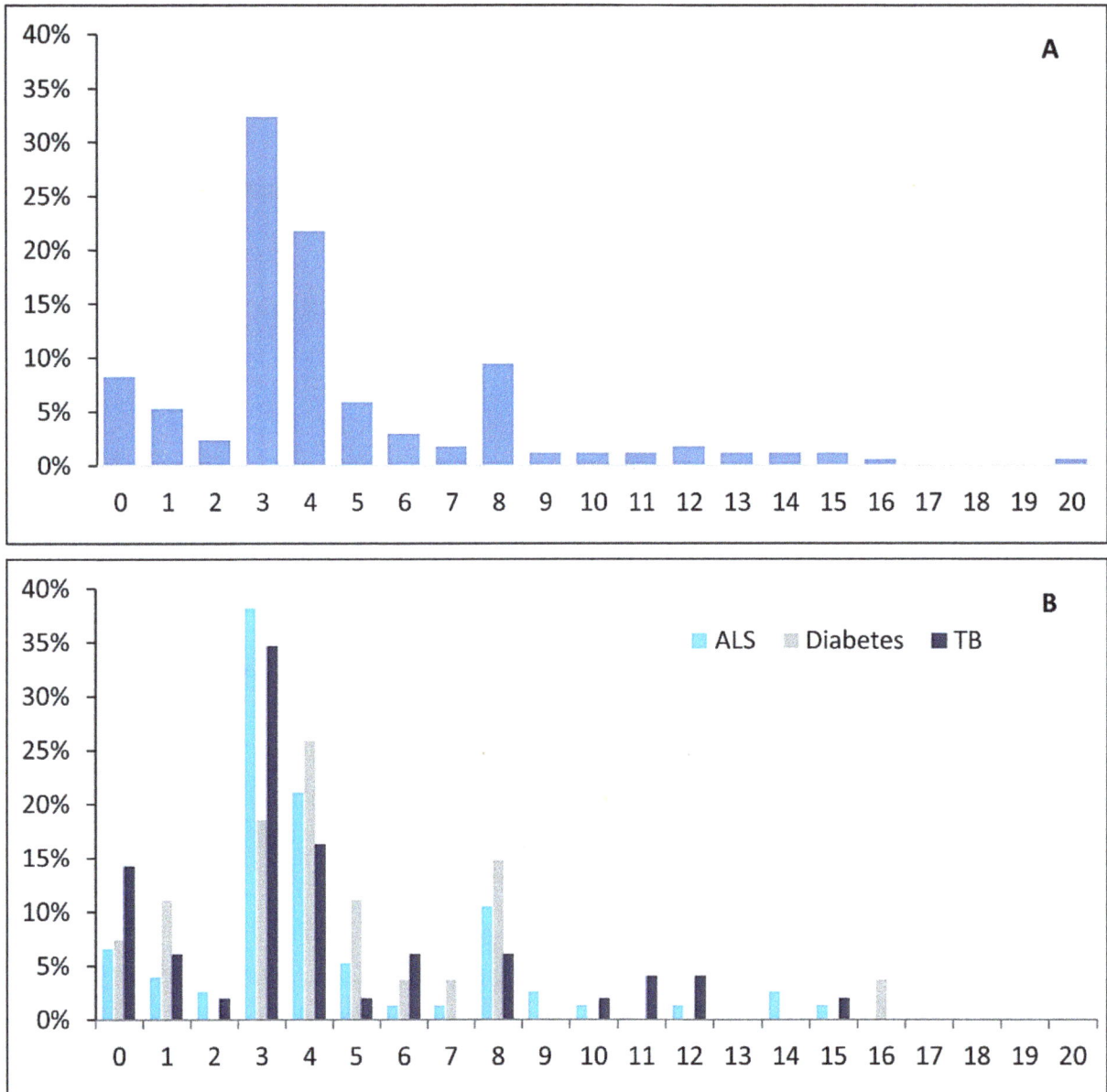

Figure 3. EXEMPLAR score distribution for the whole sample (Figure 3A; N = 170) and by field of research [Figure 3B, with 18 journals publishing studies in more than one field excluded; n(ALS) = 76; n(T1D) = 27; n(TB) = 49)]. The median score for the whole sample (N = 170) was 4 points, whereas the mean scores for ALS, T1D and TB were, respectively 4.45 (SD = 3.15), 4.52 (SD = 3.286) and 4.20 (SD = 3.54).

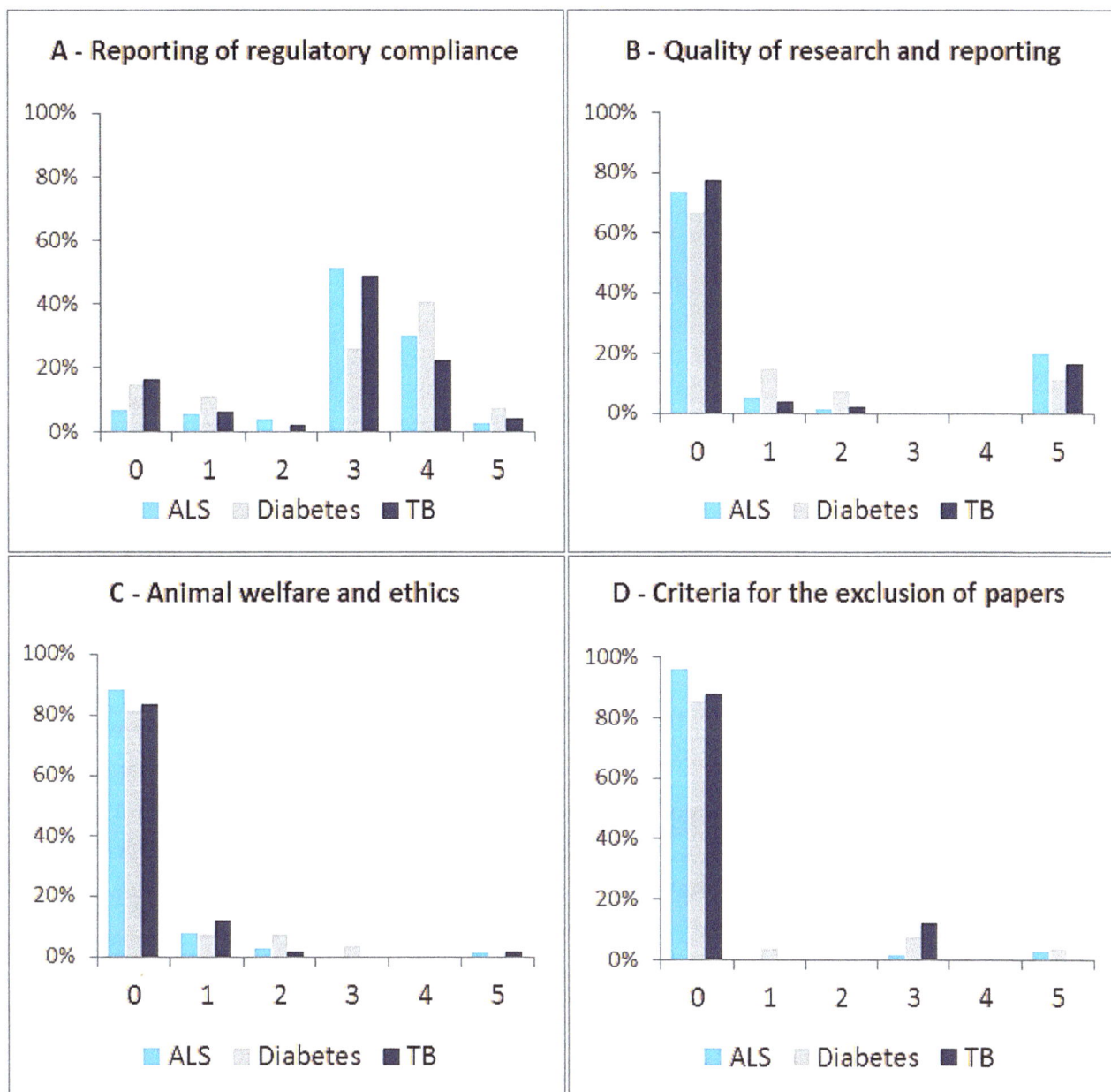

Figure 4. Scores for Categories **A**, **B**, **C** and **D**, for each. Journals publishing in more than one of the selected fields (n = 18) not shown [n(ALS) = 76; n(T1D) = 27; n(TB) = 49)].

3.3. Relationship between EXEMPLAR Score and Other Parameters

EXEMPLAR score and scores by the Osborne *et al.* scale (Figure 5) showed a positive correlation (Pearson's r = 0.623, $p < 0.001$). The sample showed a mean "Osborne score" of 2.98 points with a standard deviation of 1.28. Less than 25% of journals' scored more than three points (out of 12), and 8% of journals had a nil score by the Osborne *et al.* scale. Impact factor, country of origin, scientific category and first year of edition of scientific journals had no effect on the overall EXEMPLAR score. The model of publication (subscription *vs.* open access journals) was however shown to influence the overall EXEMPLAR score, as significantly more open access journals scored eight points or above ($\chi^2(1) = 17.87$, $p < 0.001$) than subscription based journals (Figure 6). Also, scores varied significantly between publishers ($\chi^2(53) = 96.968$, $p = 0.001$), as well as between journals from the same publisher.

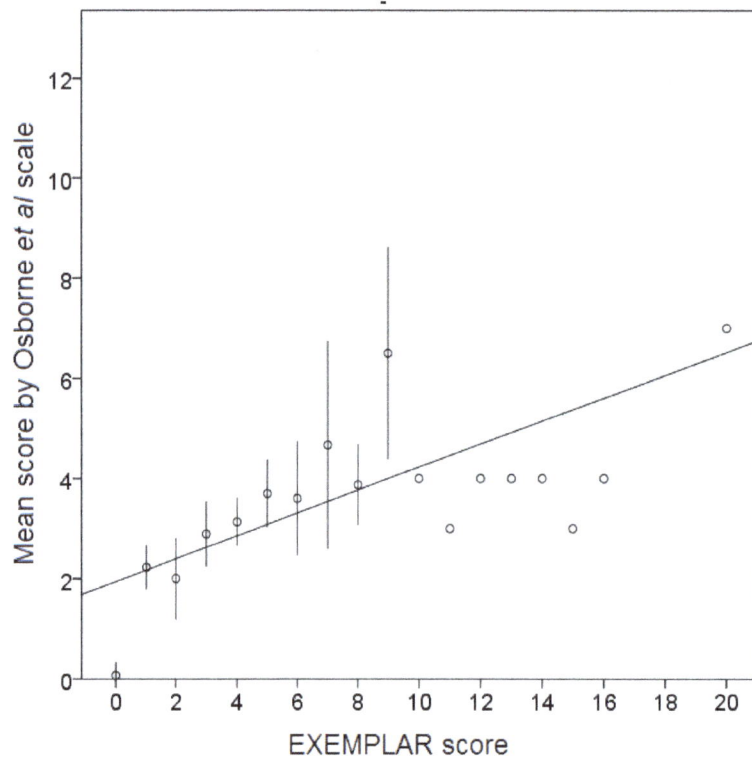

Figure 5. The mean "Osborne score" for journals with the same EXEMPLAR classification, with an overlaid best-fit regression line ($R^2 = 0.39$). Error bars represent ± 1 standard deviation of the mean for "Osborne score", for a confidence interval of 95%. No journal was classified with an EXEMPLAR score of 17, 18 or 19 points. Correlation was stronger (Pearson's $r = 0.736$), for lower scoring journals (under 10 points in the EXEMPLAR scale, corresponding to 91% of the sample).

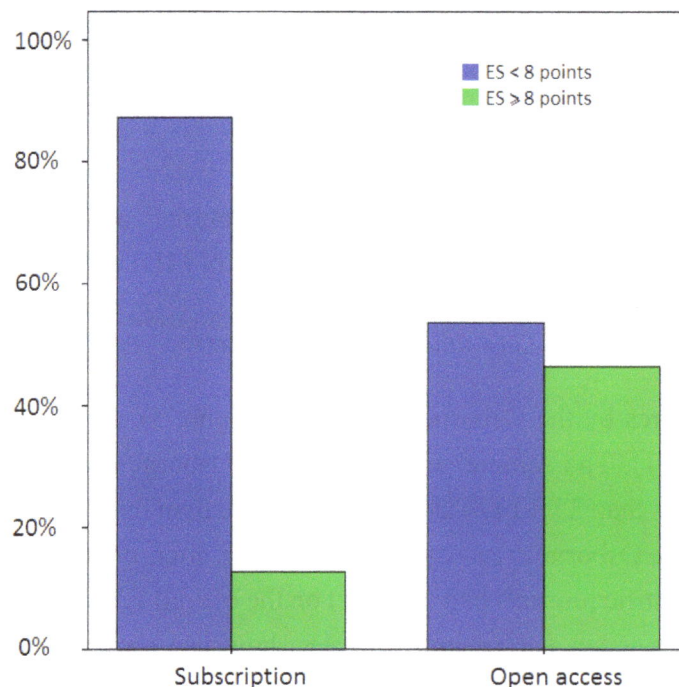

Figure 6. The proportion of open access journals with an ES ≥ 8 is significantly higher than that of subscription-based journals.

4. Discussion and Conclusions

Our results suggest a more positive scenario than previous reviews of journal policies [27–29], as some level of concern is patent by most journals in our sample requiring a statement on regulatory compliance. However, the little progress found regarding in-house policies on the ethical treatment of animals is worrisome.

Both the EXEMPLAR and 'Osborne *et al.*'s scoring of our sample paint the same overall scenario, and scores of the two classification schemes were, thus, not surprisingly, correlated. However, the EXEMPLAR allowed for a much higher differentiation between journals' policies; for any given group of journals with the same 'Osborne *et al.*' score, several EXEMPLAR scores were often given; for instance, the 94 journals scoring three points by Osborne *et al.*'s scale were classified under ten different EXEMPLAR scores, ranging between one and 15 points. The latter included the journal with the second-most comprehensive and stringent policy on animal use, namely *PLOS Genetics*, with an *EXEMPLAR score = 15:(5,5,5,0)*. Additionally, the top-scoring journal *PLOS One* [*EXEMPLAR score = 20:(5,5,5,5)*] only received six points by the 'Osborne *et al.*' classification'. These discrepancies likely result from the EXEMPLAR covering some relevant items not contemplated by Osborne *et al.*'s scale, as well as from the different weight given to some items on the overall score. Also, we consider the EXEMPLAR to be more grounded on what in the current landscape can reasonably be expected from a journal with the highest standards, whereas some of the 'Osborne *et al.*' criteria could be considered more unrealistic (e.g., expecting journals to "demand that authors 'improve on minimum standards set out in the relevant legislation") or unnecessary (for instance, no journals demanded that "investigators and all personnel who handle and use animals are appropriately trained and qualified", a likely consequence of journals assuming that only adequately trained professionals are granted licenses to work with animals).

Of all the parameters analyzed, only model of publication showed to significantly impact the overall EXEMPLAR score, which may be a consequence of open access journals being more freely accessible and hence more open to public scrutiny. This finding apparently contradicts a previous report [29] that accessibility to articles played no influence on the ethical stance of scientific journals on animal use. The latter, however, focused only on whether journals "required demonstrating adherence to any ethical guidelines", a very superficial view of ethical standards that by the EXEMPLAR scale would be solely covered by Category A. The said study also proposed that older journals were more likely to require authors to provide a statement of regulatory compliance, a claim also challenged by our data. It has also been suggested that high impact factor journals may request less details on the animal experiments they publish [24]. At least judging from what is explicitly required by journals in their instructions for authors, we have not found any evidence that such a relationship could exist.

Most journals received one or more points for Category A, for regulatory compliance, in line with previous findings that statements of compliance with animal care guidelines and ethical approval of protocols have been on the rise and are now almost universally present in biomedical papers [30,31]. However, and considering the overall poor performance of journals in the other categories, this may imply that publishers transfer their responsibilities regarding the ethical treatment and use of animals to the institutions where the studies are carried out, or its regulators. This is particularly troublesome since the mere statement of compliance to animal care guidelines, or that a given project has been approved by regulators, do not necessarily mean that said project has gone through a thorough and balanced harm-benefit (*i.e.*, "ethical") appraisal. Moreover, even if a project is indeed evaluated by a third party, principles and practice may vary greatly between different ethics committees (or equivalent), institutions or countries, as shown for instance by Plous and Herzog in 2001, who found an 80% disagreement between the decisions of different institutional animal care and use committee (IACUCs) over the same protocol [32].

From a regulatory point-of-view, project evaluation is often a "hybrid" between external (*i.e.*, legislation) and internal (by the scientific community) regulation of animal research, as it is usually a legal requirement, but on the other hand primarily carried out by scientists or others working in scientific institutions [33], which can lead to biases and conflicts of interests. Moreover, even if ethical appraisal is impartially carried out by knowledgeable and competent persons, this does not guarantee that the process is followed by any supervision or retrospective assessment, or that researchers going beyond the limits of their license are held accountable [34]. In fact, unacceptably severe studies (e.g., with death as an endpoint) may indeed be more prone to report any kind of regulatory compliance [30,31]. Despite these issues, since project approval does involve a third party to make a harm-benefit evaluation of the project, it was decided that it should have more weight on the overall score than the mere statement of compliance with norms and guidelines by authors, as these might be prompted by journal policy requirements, rather than having been in fact observed during the planning and execution of the experiments.

Although most journals had no explicit policies in place for the quality of reporting—covered by Category B—this category nonetheless obtained a higher mean score than the categories covering the ethical treatment of animals and the existence of criteria for the exclusion of papers. Indeed, 18% of journals were awarded the maximum score for this category, in virtually all of the cases for referring authors to the ARRIVE guidelines [23]. We opted to acknowledge journals for referring authors to reporting guidelines, even when compliance with said guidelines is not mandatory. The reasons behind our choice were, firstly, to be more realistic as regards to the current landscape, since only one journal in our sample—*PLOS Medicine*—made it mandatory to submit an ARRIVE checklist at the time of our analysis (*PLOS ONE* has, however, very recently changed its policies and now also requires submission of an ARRIVE checklist). Secondly, the actual enforcing of reporting guidelines relies on a clear understanding and communication between editors, reviewers and authors on this matter, which cannot be assessed by any analysis of the information made available in journals' websites.

It is encouraging that journals are increasingly referring authors to reporting guidelines. However, the level of adherence is still very low, in line with recent reports that nearly half of the editors in veterinary journals are unaware of any guidelines for reporting of animal experiments [35]. The upholding of reporting standards by scientific journals is of central importance to allow an informed interpretation of published results, as well as to allow replication of the experiments, a cornerstone of scientific research. Also, having sufficient information on the experimental protocol and results available is of central importance for systematic reviews and meta-analyses, which provide evidence of treatment effects to inform clinical research [24]. Journals requiring detailed information on experimental design and statistics can also help improve the quality of research itself, as researchers wanting to publish their results in journals with high reporting standards must consider best practice in the project planning phase. Furthermore, currently available checklists listing key parameters of sound animal research (e.g., power analysis, random assignment of animals to treatment groups or blinding of observers [36]) or animal welfare (such as cage enrichments, pain alleviation or humane endpoints) can help researchers verify whether these are in place when planning and executing an experiment [37]. Attention to experimental design and adequate statistics can also allow for using only as many animals as scientifically necessary, hence following the 3Rs principle of *reduction* [36]. Additionally, improving journals' adherence to reporting guidelines can help prevent the waste of animals' lives and resources on irreproducible—on account of insufficient information in papers—or unreliable studies skewed by unaccounted biases and methodological errors [38–41].

The high number of nil-scoring journals for Category C—"Ethical treatment of animals"—is particularly worrisome, as the ethical [42], social [8] and legal [16] acceptability of animal experiments is typically grounded on a harm-benefit balance, which not only warrants animal use to be adequately justified, but also requires that experiments cause the least possible impact on animal welfare. It is also the category that focuses more on journals' proactivity in promoting the ethical treatment of animals in research, thus becoming, as proposed by Bernard Rollin, true "guardians of the gates for animal welfare" [26]. The EXEMPLAR deliberately places a greater focus on refinement in this category, from the assumption that it is more reasonable to expect that editors and reviewers are willing—and have the needed expertise—to deal with the question of *how* studies submitted for publication were carried out than to judge if these should have rather been carried out by non-animal methods in the first place.

There are, however, limitations to what can be ascertained about how animals are treated from what researchers report, but editors and reviewers with reasons to question animal welfare standards should be able to ask authors the needed information to clarify this matter and determine if indeed animal suffering was excessive or unjustified. Furthermore, there is only so much that can be asked of reviewers, who for each paper they are asked to review have to carry out a specialized and unpaid work in a short period of time [43]. Also, the reviewers' main task is usually to appraise manuscripts from a scientific point-of-view, being thus chosen for their expertise on a given field, rather than on ethics and animal welfare. These may hence lack the knowledge—and sometimes even the empathy—needed to adequately assess whether "all efforts were made to minimize suffering" (the standard, almost *cliché*, statement that can often be found in papers reporting unacceptably severe studies), or critically evaluate if the soundness and value of the study justify the cost borne by animals. Hence, editors' duty must go beyond merely requiring a statement of compliance with local regulations [28,34,44].

The overwhelming majority of journals had no explicit statement on the exclusion of manuscripts for the unethical treatment of animals, covered by Category D. The absence of a statement demanding compliance with journal policies for manuscript acceptance does not necessarily imply that editors do not enforce them, but the fact that no measurable progress in the quality of reporting has been observed in journals endorsing the ARRIVE guidelines [45] raises the question of how effective journal policies are in promoting best practice in other aspects of animal research, as well, including those measured by the EXEMPLAR scale.

The conclusions that can be drawn from the data presented here have some limitations. Firstly, our sample was retrieved from a list of papers written in English, leaving out several scientific journals publishing in other languages such as Spanish, Portuguese, Mandarin or Russian, to name a few. Also, the EXEMPLAR scale was designed to classify explicitly stated journal policies, so scores may thus reflect "good intentions" rather than actual attitudes and practice by editors and reviewers. On the other hand, there might also be cases in which the opposite is true, as editors and reviewers who are sensitive to scientific and ethical issues on animal use may have their own set of criteria and apply them accordingly, regardless of explicitly stated journal policies. There may also be an inherent bias in our journal selection process, which aimed for high representativity of the selected fields (as the journals in the sample represent 75%, 73% and 72% of all ALS, T1D and TB papers published between 2011 and 2013, respectively) but on the other hand potentially limiting the extent to which these results can be extrapolated to the whole population of biomedical journals. There is, however, considerable diversity between the selected fields, and all major publishers were represented, as well as generalist journals, such as *PLOS ONE*, *Nature*, *PNAS* or the *EMBO journal*, among others. Furthermore, of all the journals retrieved from the original search results, only one was excluded for not publishing animal studies.

The disappointingly low scores found in our sample led us to consider the possibility that the EXEMPLAR could be setting unachievable standards. While a few high-scoring journals were found in our sample, we nevertheless analyzed a selection of five journals outside our original sample, reputed for their high standards regarding the ethical treatment of animals in research. These included two journals on laboratory animal science—*JAALAS* [EXEMPLAR =**16**:(2,5,5,4)] and *Laboratory Animals* [EXEMPLAR = **18**:(5,5,5,3)]—two others on animal welfare—*Animal Welfare* [EXEMPLAR= **15**:(4,5,3,3) and *Journal of Applied Animal Welfare* [EXEMPLAR=**12**:(2,2,5,3)]—and also MDPI's *Animals* [EXEMPLAR = **15**:(5,5,5,3). These scores attest to the construct validity of the EXEMPLAR scale (*i.e.*, the degree to which it the scale measures what it intends to be measuring), as it allowed identifying quantitatively the (subjectively perceived) high standards of this selection of journals.

Overall, our data suggest there is still much to be done as regards the attention given by biomedical journals to the scientific and ethical issues underlying animal research. The main challenge will be finding how to make journal policies promote best practice, when most journals have failed [45] to ensure adherence to reasonable [44] principles of transparency and rigorous reporting, despite the set of guidelines and checklists now available for this purpose. A checklist for journal policies on animal welfare could hence also fail to have a meaningful impact in laboratory animals' lives, because unlike reporting guidelines—that can be more broadly adopted—defining animal welfare requirements warrants a case-by-case approach, depending on the type of model used, choice of procedures and the scientific objectives. This may partially explain why compliance with regulations is a requirement for most journals, while having in-house policies in place on the ethical treatment of animals is not.

In conclusion, a re-evaluation of scientific journals' current policies, as well as an improvement in the communication between editors and reviewers to implement such policies is of the essence [44]. A discussion of these results and of the standards upheld by the EXEMPLAR may be a good starting point.

Acknowledgments

The authors would wish to thank I. Anna S. Olsson for valuable comments on the EXEMPLAR Scale and on an earlier version of the present article, and Nicola J. Osborne for her valuable input on the EXEMPLAR scale. Nuno Henrique Franco is the recipient of a post-doctoral grant (reference SFRH/BPD/85978/2012) by the Portuguese Foundation for Science and Technology (FCT).

Author Contributions

NHF conceived and designed the experiments; ARM performed the experiments; ARM and NHF analyzed the data; ARM and NHF wrote the paper.

Conflicts of Interest

The authors declare no conflict of interest.

References

1. Franco, N.H. Animal experiments in biomedical research: A historical perspective. *Animals* **2013**, *3*, 238–273.

2. Hagelin, J.; Carlsson, H.-E.; Hau, J. An overview of surveys on how people view animal experimentation: Some factors that may influence the outcome. *Public Underst. Sci.* **2003**, *12*, 67–81.

3. Ormandy, E.H.; Schuppli, C.A.; Weary, D.M. Public attitudes toward the use of animals in research: Effects of invasiveness, genetic modification and regulation. *Anthrozoos: Multidiscip. J. Interact. People Anim.* **2013**, *26*, 165–184.

4. European Commission. Results of Questionnaire for the General Public on the Revision of Directive 86/609/EEC on the Protection of Animals Used for Experimental and Other Scientific Purposes. Available online: http://ec.europa.eu/environment/chemicals/lab_animals/pdf/results_citizens.pdf (accessed on 12 November 2014).

5. Lund, T.B.; Sørensen, T.I.A.; Olsson, I.A.S.; Hansen, A.K.; Sandøe, P. Is it acceptable to use animals to model obese humans? A critical discussion of two arguments against the use of animals in obesity research. *J. Med. Ethics* **2014**, *40*, 320–324.

6. Aldhous, P.; Coghlan, A.; Copley, J. Animal experiments—Where do you draw the line?: Let the people speak. *New Sci.* **1999**, *162*, 26–31.

7. Worcester, R.M. Science and society: What scientists and the public can learn from each other. *Proc. R. Inst.* **2001**, *71*, 97–160.

8. Lund, T.B.; Mørkbak, M.R.; Lassen, J.; Sandøe, P. Painful dilemmas: A study of the way the public's assessment of animal research balances costs to animals against human benefits. *Public Underst. Sci.* **2014**, *23*, 428–444.

9. TNS Opinion & Social. *Special Eurobarometer 340/Wave 73.1: Science and Technology.* Brussels; Directorate General Research, European Commission. **2010**

10. Pifer, L.; Shimizu, K.; Pifer, R. Public attitudes toward animal research: Some international comparisons. *Soc. Anim.* **1994**, *2*, 95–113.

11. Serpell, J.A. Factors influencing human attitudes to animals and their welfare. *Anim. Welf.* **2004**, *13*, S145–S152.

12. Holmberg, T.; Ideland, M. Secrets and lies: "Selective openness" in the apparatus of animal experimentation. *Public Underst. Sci.* **2012**, *21*, 354–368.

13. Von Roten, F.C. Public perceptions of animal experimentation across Europe. *Public Underst. Sci.* **2012**, doi: 10.1177/0963662511428045.

14. Russell, W.M.S.; Burch, R.L. *The Principles of Humane Experimental Technique*; Methuen & Co. Ltd: London, UK, 1959.

15. Festing, S.; Wilkinson, R. The ethics of animal research. *EMBO Rep.* **2007**, *8*, 526–530.

16. Louhimies, S. Eu directive 2010/63/eu: "Implementing the three rs through policy". *ALTEX Proc.* **2012**, *1*, 27–33.

17. Dixon-Woods, M.; Ashcroft, R. Regulation and the social licence for medical research. *Med. Health Care Philos.* **2008**, *11*, 381–391.

18. Varga, O.; Hansen, A.K.; Sandoe, P.; Olsson, I.A.S. Improving transparency and ethical accountability in animal studies. *Embo Rep.* **2010**, *11*, 500–503.

19. Wells, D.J. Animal welfare and the 3rs in european biomedical research. *Ann. N.Y. Acad. Sci.* **2011**, *1245*, 14–16.

20. Jennings, M.; Smith, J.A. Ethical review of animal experiments: Current practice and future directions. *ALTEX Proc.* **2012**, *1*, 275–279.

21. Forni, M. Laboratory animal science: A resource to improve the quality of science. *Vet. Res. Commun.* **2007**, *31*, 43–47.

22. Smaje, L.H.; Smith, J.A.; Combes, R.D.; Ewbank, R.; Gregory, J.A.; Jennings, M.; Moore, G.J.; Morton, D.B. Advancing refinement of laboratory animal use. *Lab. Anim.* **1998**, *32*, 137–142.

23. Kilkenny, C.; Browne, W.J.; Cuthill, I.C.; Emerson, M.; Altman, D.G. Improving bioscience research reporting: The arrive guidelines for reporting animal research. *PLoS Biol.* **2010**, *8*, e1000412.

24. Hooijmans, C.R.; Leenaars, M.; Ritskes-Hoitinga, M. A gold standard publication checklist to improve the quality of animal studies, to fully integrate the three rs, and to make systematic reviews more feasible. *ATLA-Altern. Lab. Anim.* **2010**, 38, 167-182.

25. Basel Declaration Society. Basel declaration: A call for more trust, transparency and communication on animal research. In *Research at a Crossroads*; Basel Declaration Society: Basel, Switzerland, **2010**.

26. Rollin, B.E. Animal research, animal welfare, and the three Rs. Available online: http://jpsl.org/archives/animal-research-animal-welfare-and-three-rs/ (accessed on 3 November 2014).

27. Osborne, N.J.; Phillips, B.J.; Westwood, K. Journal editorial policies as a driver for change—Animal welfare and the 3Rs. In *New Paradigms In Laboratory Animal Science*, Proceedings of the Eleventh FELASA Symposium and the 40th Scand-LAS Symposium, Helsinki, Finland, 14–17 June 2010; FELASA: Helsinki, Finland, 2011, pp. 18–23.

28. Osborne, N.J.; Payne, D.; Newman, M.L. Journal editorial policies, animal welfare, and the 3Rs. *Am. J. Bioeth.* **2009**, *9*, 55–59.

29. Rands, S., Ethical policies on animal experiments are not compromised by whether a journal is freely accessible or charges for publication. *Animal* **2009**, *3*, 1591–1595.

30. Franco, N.H.; Olsson, I. "How sick must your mouse be?"—An analysis of the use of animal models in huntington's disease research. *ATLA* **2012**, *40*, 271–283.

31. Franco, N.H.; Correia-Neves, M.; Olsson, I.A.S. Animal welfare in studies on murine tuberculosis: Assessing progress over a 12-year period and the need for further improvement. *PLOS ONE* **2012**, *7*, e47723.

32. Plous, S.; Herzog, H. Animal research. Reliability of protocol reviews for animal research. *Science* **2001**, *293*, 608–609.

33. Varga, O.; Olsson, I.A.S. 6.2. Animal ethics committees: Different regions—Imilar tasks and difficulties?—European union. In *Ethical Aspects of Animal Research—Life in the Lab*; Gjerris, M., Olsson, I.A.S., Röcklinsberg, H., Eds.; Springer: in press.

34. Franco, N.H.; Olsson, I. Is the ethical appraisal of protocols enough to ensure best practice in animal research? *ATLA* **2013**, *41*, P5–P7.

35. Grindlay, D.J.; Dean, R.S.; Christopher, M.M.; Brennan, M.L. A survey of the awareness, knowledge, policies and views of veterinary journal editors-in-chief on reporting guidelines for publication of research. *BMC Vet. Res.* **2014**, *10*, 10.

36. Festing, M.F.; Altman, D.G. Guidelines for the design and statistical analysis of experiments using laboratory animals. *ILAR J.* **2002**, *43*, 244–258.

37. Hooijmans, C.R.; de Vries, R.; Leenaars, M.; Curfs, J.; Ritskes-Hoitinga, M. Improving planning, design, reporting and scientific quality of animal experiments by using the gold standard publication checklist, in addition to the arrive guidelines. *Br. J. Pharmacol.* **2011**, *162*, 1259–1260.

38. Van der Worp, H.B.; Howells, D.W.; Sena, E.S.; Porritt, M.J.; Rewell, S.; O'Collins, V.; Macleod, M.R. Can animal models of disease reliably inform human studies? *PLOS Med.* **2010**, *7*, e1000245.

39. Landis, S.C.; Amara, S.G.; Asadullah, K.; Austin, C.P.; Blumenstein, R.; Bradley, E.W.; Crystal, R.G.; Darnell, R.B.; Ferrante, R.J.; Fillit, H.; *et al.* A call for transparent reporting to optimize the predictive value of preclinical research. *Nature* **2012**, *490*, 187–191.

40. Kilkenny, C.; Parsons, N.; Kadyszewski, E.; Festing, M.F.; Cuthill, I.C.; Fry, D.; Hutton, J.; Altman, D.G. Survey of the quality of experimental design, statistical analysis and reporting of research using animals. *PLOS ONE* **2009**, *4*, e7824.

41. Eisen, J.A.; Ganley, E.; MacCallum, C.J. Open science and reporting animal studies: Who's accountable? *PLOS Biol.* **2014**, *12*, e1001757.

42. Olsson, I.A.S.; Robinson, P.; Sandøe, P. Ethics of animal research. *Handb. Lab. Anim. Sci.* **2011**, *1*, 21–35.

43. Hirst, A.; Altman, D.G. Are peer reviewers encouraged to use reporting guidelines? A survey of 116 health research journals. *PLOS ONE* **2012**, *7*, e35621.

44. Galley, H.F. Mice, men, and medicine. *Br. J. Anaesth.* **2010**, *105*, 396–400.

45. Baker, D.; Lidster, K.; Sottomayor, A.; Amor, S. Two years later: Journals are not yet enforcing the arrive guidelines on reporting standards for pre-clinical animal studies. *PLOS Biol.* **2014**, *12*, e1001756.

8

The Effects of Fiber Inclusion on Pet Food Sensory Characteristics and Palatability

Kadri Koppel [1],*, Mariana Monti [2], Michael Gibson [3], Sajid Alavi [3], Brizio Di Donfrancesco [1] and Aulus Cavalieri Carciofi [2]

[1] Sensory Analysis Center, Department of Human Nutrition, Kansas State University, 1310 Research Park Drive, Manhattan, KS 66502, USA; E-Mail: briziod@ksu.edu

[2] Department of Veterinary Clinic and Surgery, College of Agricultural and Veterinarian Sciences, São Paulo State University (UNESP), Via de Acesso Prof. Paulo Donato Castellane, s/n, Jaboticabal, SP 14.884-900, Brazil; E-Mails: mariana_814@hotmail.com (M.M.); aulus.carciofi@gmail.com (A.C.)

[3] Department of Grain Science and Industry, Kansas State University, Manhattan, KS 66506, USA; E-Mails: michael.gibson171@gmail.com (M.G.); salavi@ksu.edu (S.A.)

* Author to whom correspondence should be addressed; E-Mail: kadri@ksu.edu.

Academic Editor: Marina von Keyserling

Simple Summary: The results from this research indicate that fibers have an effect on extruded pet food texture and palatability. These results may help pet food companies select ingredients for successful product formulations.

Abstract: The objectives of this study were to determine (a) the influence of fiber on the sensory characteristics of dry dog foods; (b) differences of coated and uncoated kibbles for aroma and flavor characteristics; (c) palatability of these dry dog foods; and (d) potential associations between palatability and sensory attributes. A total of eight fiber treatments were manufactured: a control (no fiber addition), guava fiber (3%, 6%, and 12%), sugar cane fiber (9%; large and small particle size), and wheat bran fiber (32%; large and small particle size). The results indicated significant effects of fibers on both flavor and texture properties of the samples. Bitter taste and iron and stale aftertaste were examples of flavor attributes that differed with treatment, with highest intensity observed for 12% guava fiber and small particle size sugar cane fiber treatments. Fracturability and initial crispness attributes were lowest for the sugar cane fiber treatments. Flavor of all treatments changed after coating with a palatant, increasing in toasted, brothy, and grainy attributes. The coating also had a masking effect on aroma attributes such as stale, flavor attributes such as iron and bitter taste, and appearance attributes such as porosity. Palatability testing results indicated that the control treatment was preferred over the sugar cane or the wheat bran treatment. The treatment with large sugarcane fiber particles was preferred over the treatment with small particles, while both of the wheat bran treatments were eaten at a similar level. Descriptive sensory analysis data, especially textural attributes, were useful in pinpointing the underlying characteristics and were considered to be reasons that may influence palatability of dog foods manufactured with inclusion of different fibers.

Keywords: dog food; extruded; fiber; palatability, sensory analysis

---

1. Introduction

Pet foods are manufactured with a myriad of ingredients. Mimicking human food trends, these ingredients are often of novel origin. Sensory properties of pet food products may be influenced by types of ingredients used in the formulation, added palatants, and processing factors used. Protein, grain, and fiber sources can influence the appearance, aroma, flavor and texture of extruded dog food. To understand the sensory characteristics of products manufactured with fibers of different source, eight extruded products were evaluated in this study.

Fibers are structural carbohydrates, mainly originating from plant cell walls. The energy available from fibers is limited, and because of this, fibers may be good ingredients in reduced energy diets [1]. In addition it has been found that fibers in combination with proteins help regulate satiety levels in dogs [2]. Furthermore, fibers may help regulate the digestive process and the glycemic response in dogs and cats [3,4]. Depending on the fiber type and consumed amount, different effects on nutrient digestibility and fecal formation can be promoted [4].

Previous studies have described dietary fiber effects on sensory properties of different types of foods. The different sources and amounts of dietary fibers have an effect on the texture of extruded products due to the interaction with starch [5]. The increase of insoluble fiber (mainly wheat bran) was shown to increase the hardness of extruded cereals because of reduced expansion volumes and increased density [5]. Dietary fibers enrichment in bread showed a reduction of loaf volume, with the crumbs having higher firmness and a darker appearance [6]. Other studies on bread showed that a higher content of dietary fibers resulted in smaller cells in the crumb, which in turn resulted in a more dense appearance [7]. Popov-Ralić et al. [8] observed that different fiber content in cookies mostly impacted the appearance of the products, in particular the color.

Most common sources of fiber in pet foods are beet pulp and cellulose. Corn fiber, fruit fibers, rice bran, and whole grains are some of the other fiber sources available for use in pet foods [3]. Full-fat rice bran was tested for palatability and digestibility in pet foods by Pacheco et al. [9]. These authors found that rice bran could be used in pet foods, but at no more than a 20% inclusion rate. Sa et al. [10] studied an enzyme treatment effect on dog foods manufactured with wheat bran. These authors found that the enzymes did not have an effect on digestibility, but wheat bran addition resulted in a larger amount of fecal matter being produced.

Understanding pet food palatability issues is not an easy task as the test animals lack the necessary linguistic capabilities. Descriptive sensory analysis by trained human panelists may provide insight into pet food palatability [11]. Descriptive sensory analysis will not tell us how the food tastes for the target species, such as dogs or cats, but will further our understanding regarding the sensory properties of the products. Sensory studies on pet foods have found that dry dog foods are generally complex products that vary in appearance, aroma, flavor, and texture [12,13]. A study that compared baked and extruded dog foods found that the pet food textures resulting from these cooking methods were significantly different [14]. However, so far no studies have been found that compare the sensory properties of pet foods to palatability or animal liking of the foods. The primary hypothesis of this study is that fiber source has an effect on sensory characteristics such as flavor and texture properties and palatability of pet foods.

The objectives of this study were to determine the following characteristics for dry dog foods formulated with a significant proportion of dietary fiber: (a) the effect of fiber on the sensory characteristics; (b) differences between coated and uncoated kibbles for aroma and flavor characteristics; (c) palatability of selected coated treatments; and (d) potential associations between palatability and sensory flavor and texture attributes.

2. Experimental Section

2.1. Diet Formulation

A basal diet containing maize and poultry by-product meal was formulated for adult dog maintenance according to the European Pet Food Industry Federation nutritional guidelines for complete and complementary pet food for cats and dogs [15]. Different types of fiber, sourced from Dilumix (Leme, Sao Paulo, Brazil), were added to this basal diet to create eight treatments as described in Table 1: control, with no fiber addition (CO); guava fruit fiber (67% insoluble dietary fiber, less than 1% soluble fiber) at the inclusion levels of 3%, 6%, and 12% (GF3, GF6, and GF12, respectively); sugarcane fiber (90% insoluble dietary fiber, less than 1% soluble fiber) with large particle size (SC1) and small particle size (SC2; Vit2be Fiber; inclusion level 9% for both treatments); and wheat bran fiber (32% insoluble dietary fiber, 1.5% soluble fiber) with large particle size (WB1) and small particle size (WB2). Ingredients were previously analyzed and the diets containing 12% guava fiber (GF12), sugarcane fiber (SC1 and SC2) and wheat bran (WB1 and WB2) were balanced to have 16% of total dietary fiber, which is a level typically used in commercial high-fiber dog diets. All fibers were added by replacing corn.

2.2. Grinding and Mixing

The ingredients, with the exception of fiber sources, were weighed, mixed, and ground using a hammer mill fitted with a screen size of 0.8 mm (Sistema Tigre de Mistura e Moagem, Tigre, Sao Paulo, Brazil). Fiber sources were provided already ground to desired particle sizes by the supplier (Dilumix, Leme, SP, Brazil): guava fiber—213 μm; large sugarcane fiber—395 μm; small sugar cane fiber—197 μm;

large wheat bran—345 µm; small wheat bran—143 µm. These sizes were determined using laser diffraction particle size analysis [16]. The other ingredients and fiber sources were then mixed, compounding the final diet.

Table 1. Treatment ingredients and nutritional composition, % *.

Ingredients, %	CO	GF3	GF6	GF12	SC1	SC2	WB1	WB2
Corn grain	57.9	54.6	51.2	44.6	47.5	47.5	30.4	30.4
Chicken byproduct meal	31.3	31.6	31.8	32.3	32.6	32.6	26.1	26.1
Chicken Fat	7.0	7.0	7.3	7.4	7.2	7.2	7.6	7.6
Guava Fiber	0.0	3.0	6.0	12.0	0.0	0.0	0.0	0.0
Sugar Cane Fiber	0.0	0.0	0.0	0.0	9.0	9.0	0.0	0.0
Wheat Bran	0.0	0.0	0.0	0.0	0.0	0.0	32.0	32.0
Fish oil	0.15	0.15	0.15	0.15	0.15	0.15	0.15	0.15
Palatant	2	2	2	2	2	2	2	2
NaCl	0.5	0.5	0.5	0.5	0.5	0.5	0.65	0.65
KCl	0.5	0.5	0.5	0.5	0.5	0.5	0.5	0.5
Vitamin and Mineral mix	0.3	0.3	0.3	0.3	0.3	0.3	0.3	0.3
Choline Chloride	0.2	0.2	0.2	0.2	0.2	0.2	0.2	0.2
Mold inhibitor agent	0.1	0.1	0.1	0.1	0.1	0.1	0.1	0.1
Antioxidant agent	0.04	0.04	0.04	0.04	0.04	0.04	0.04	0.04
Nutritional Composition in the final product (on DM-basis)								
Crude Protein	29.1	28.8	28.4	28.5	29.4	29.5	28.0	28.2
Crude Fat	15.3	15.9	15.2	14.6	15.0	14.7	14.5	15.5
Ash	6.4	6.0	7.0	6.1	5.8	6.2	6.5	6.4
Crude Fiber	1.9	3.0	3.9	4.7	4.6	4.2	3.1	3.7
Dietary fiber	8.0	9.9	11.9	15.7	16,1	16.3	16.9	16.7
Starch	40.2	38.7	35.7	34.6	35.6	34.8	32.4	32.4
Moisture	5.9	6.8	6.0	7.3	5.4	5.3	5.6	5.5

* CO-Control, GF3—3% guava fiber, GF6—6% guava fiber, GF12—12% guava fiber, SC1—sugar cane fiber large grind, SC2—sugar cane fiber small grind, WB1—wheat bran fiber, large grind, WB2—wheat bran fiber, small grind.

2.3. Extrusion

The diets were extruded in a single screw extruder (MEX 250, Mazoni, Campinas, Brazil), with a processing capacity of 250 kg/h. Each food was processed separately on two different days for replicates. The processing conditions were not changed for any treatment in order to isolate the influence of fiber. Four samples were collected per diet each day and pooled. Pooled samples from both days were combined into one batch per diet for the sensory and palatability studies. For each diet, suitable amounts of samples were selected for coating for palatability and sensory tests from the same consolidated batch as the uncoated samples. A pre-conditioner was used to treat the diets with steam and water prior to extrusion. The pre-conditioner residence time was approximately 3.5 min, and downspout temperature was 82.2–85.7 °C. The extruder screw speed was 465 rpm, and the die open area was 15.9 mm^2/ton/h. Extruder die temperature ranged between 118.7–130.3 °C and die pressure between 52.45–70.6 bar. After extrusion, the kibbles were dried in a forced air dryer at 105 °C for 30 minutes. The dried kibbles were coated in a tumble system, receiving first the poultry fat and then the commercial palatant D'TECH 6L (SPF, Descalvado, São Paulo, Brazil) at 2% of the ingredients. The fish oil in the formulation was mixed with dry ingredients before extrusion.

2.4. Descriptive Sensory Analysis

2.4.1. Panelists

Five highly trained panelists from the Sensory Analysis Center, Kansas State University (Manhattan, KS, USA) participated in this study. All of the panelists had completed 120 h of general descriptive analysis training with a variety of food products. The training included techniques and practice in attribute identification, terminology development, and intensity scoring. Each of the panelists had more than 1000 h of testing experience with a variety of food products. For this project, the panelists received further orientation on dried dog food using samples that may or may not be included in the study. Panels of similar size and training have been reported in other recent research [8–10].

2.4.2. Sample Presentation and Evaluation

The panelists evaluated both uncoated (no poultry fat and no palatant added) and coated (poultry fat and palatant added) kibbles to determine the effect of coating and palatant on kibble flavor.

Evaluation of uncoated kibbles (n = 8: CO, SC1, SC2, WB1, WB2, GF3, GF6, and GF12) was conducted during seven 1.5 h sessions. Evaluation of coated kibbles (n = 5: CO, SC1, SC2, WB1, and WB2) was conducted during five 1.5 h sessions.

Each sample was served in a ~100 mL plastic cup for appearance, texture, and flavor evaluation, and in a medium snifter covered with a watch glass for the evaluation of aroma. The amount of product in the snifter was 3 g. Samples were prepared 30 min prior to the testing and were coded with three-digit random numbers.

All of the uncoated samples were evaluated in a randomized order in duplicate for appearance, texture, flavor, and aroma using attributes selected from a lexicon developed for this product category by Di Donfrancesco *et al.* [12] and used by Koppel *et al.* [13]. Barnyard, brothy, toasted, grain, vitamin, stale, egg, oxidized oil, cardboard, liver, fish, metallic, and dusty/earthy aroma and flavor were evaluated in all samples. In addition sour, salty, sweet, and bitter taste and aftertaste and barnyard, vitamin, stale, oxidized oil, cardboard, liver, fish, and metallic aftertaste attributes were evaluated. Brown color intensity, porous, grainy, flecks (yes/no), and fibrous appearance characteristics and cohesiveness of mass, fracturability, hardness, initial crispness, fibrous and gritty texture attributes were evaluated. A total of two 1.5 h sessions were held for orientation purposes and five 1.5 h sessions for the evaluation phase of the samples.

The coated samples (n = 5) were evaluated in a randomized order in duplicate for aroma, flavor, and appearance attributes only. The appearance attributes evaluated were: brown, porous, grainy, fibrous, and flecks. The aroma attributes were: barnyard, brothy, toasted, grain, vitamin, egg, sour aromatics, oxidized oil, cardboard, dusty/earthy, iron, and hay-like. The flavor attributes were: barnyard, broth, toasted, grain, vitamin, egg, sour, salt, bitter, sweet, oxidized oil, cardboard, liver, fish, dusty/earthy, metallic, iron, and hay-like. A total of two 1.5 h sessions were held for orientation purposes and three 1.5 h sessions for the evaluation phase of the coated samples.

For the evaluation, a numeric scale of 0–15 with 0.5 increments where 0 represented none and 15 extremely high was applied to each attribute to provide a measure of intensity. Each panelist individually assigned intensities to the attributes present in the sample according to their perception of the appearance, aroma, flavor, and texture references included in the lexicon. The panelists were provided with a definition sheet with the list of attributes and their definitions as well as reference materials for each attribute according to Di Donfrancesco et al. [12].

The panelists were asked to chew one kibble for flavor and texture evaluation. The panelists were instructed to expectorate samples after evaluation. Panelists were provided with apple slices, unsalted crackers, purified water, and toothbrushes for palate cleansing in between the evaluations. The testing room was at 21 ± 1 °C and $55\% \pm 5\%$ relative humidity.

2.5. Palatability Testing

Palatability Testing Procedure

The tests were performed in Panelis, Diana Group (Descalvado, São Paulo, Brazil). Palatability was measured for the five fiber treatments (CO, SC1, SC2, WB1, and WB2) and with the coated kibbles only, using the two-pan method on two meals in one day, each test with 38 dogs in individual kennels [17]. The combinations of the samples were CO × SC1, CO × WB1, SC1 × SC2, and WB1 × WB2. In the morning after a 12 h fast the dogs received two pans, each containing one of the experimental foods, and were allowed to eat for 30 min. The position of the food pans was alternated at the evening meal. The amount of food offered in each pan surpassed the consumption capacity of the animal to ensure there would be leftovers to measure. After 30 min the pans were removed, the remains weighed and consumption rate was calculated (Equation (1)). Due to the large differences in body weights the results were calculated as relative consumption of each diet, and the mean intake of the two meals for each dog was compared.

$$Relative\ consumption\ (\%) = \frac{Food\ A\ consumption}{Food\ A\ consumption + Food\ B\ consumption} \times 100 \qquad (1)$$

2.6. Data Analysis

Significant differences ($p < 0.05$) among the uncoated kibble treatments and coated kibble treatments sensory properties were determined using SAS Glimmix procedure and Fisher's protected Least Significant Difference (LSD) (Version 9.3, SAS Institute Inc., Cary, NC, USA). Principal Components Analysis was conducted for the significantly different appearance, texture, aroma, and flavor attributes of Control, WB1, WB2, SC1, and SC2 using XLStat version 2014.1.08 (Addinsoft, New York, NY, USA). Dog palatability data were statistically evaluated using Analysis of Variance (ANOVA), using the SAS software (Version 9.3, SAS Institute Inc.).

3. Results and Discussion

3.1. Descriptive Sensory Analysis

3.1.1 Uncoated Treatments

The main contributing attributes to aroma for the uncoated treatments were barnyard, toasted, grainy, stale, and cardboard [18]. These attributes were higher in intensity than other attributes, but were not necessarily different among treatments. The main contributing attributes to flavor and taste for these dog foods were barnyard, toasted, grainy, vitamin, stale, sour, salty, bitter, dusty/earthy, oxidized oil, cardboard, liver, and metallic. The highest intensity was noted for bitter taste and aftertaste (averages 6.70–8.90).

The uncoated treatments were not significantly different ($p > 0.05$) in brown color, cohesiveness of mass, hardness, vitamin aftertaste, sour aftertaste, salty aftertaste, cardboard aftertaste, liver aftertaste, metallic aftertaste, barnyard flavor, broth flavor, grain flavor, vitamin flavor, sour taste, salty taste, sweet taste, cardboard flavor, liver flavor, fish flavor, metallic flavor, iron flavor, barnyard aroma, broth aroma, toasted aroma, grainy aroma, vitamin aroma, stale aroma, eggy aroma, cardboard aroma, liver aroma, fishy aroma, or iron aroma.

Table 2. Average texture, appearance, aroma, flavor, and aftertaste attributes intensity scores for uncoated treatments. Significantly different attributes showed only ($p < 0.05$).

Attribute	Treatment							
	CO	GF3	GF6	GF12	SC1	SC2	WB1	WB2
Fracturability	7.03 [a]	6.60 [ab]	6.73 [ab]	6.37 [bc]	5.67 [d]	5.63 [d]	7.17 [a]	5.90 [cd]
Initial Crispness	10.47 [a]	10.47 [a]	10.43 [a]	9.33 [b]	8.87 [bc]	8.73 [c]	10.33 [a]	9.17 [bc]
Fibrous	1.63 [de]	3.03 [bc]	0.70 [e]	2.07 [cd]	9.20 [a]	4.07 [b]	1.93 [cde]	3.10 [bc]
Gritty	4.23 [ab]	4.23 [ab]	4.87 [a]	4.03 [b]	3.37 [c]	4.13 [b]	3.97 [bc]	3.87 [bc]
Porous Appearance	5.00 [bc]	5.27 [abc]	6.13 [a]	5.80 [ab]	4.60 [c]	2.93 [d]	6.17 [a]	6.23 [a]
Grainy Appearance	2.00 [bcd]	2.10 [bc]	2.60 [ab]	1.93 [cd]	2.90 [a]	1.47 [d]	2.13 [bc]	1.90 [cd]
Fibrous Appearance	1.10 [c]	1.00 [c]	0.60 [c]	1.07 [c]	6.17 [a]	2.40 [b]	0.80 [c]	1.30 [c]
Oxidized Oil Aroma	2.13 [ab]	1.87 [b]	2.37 [a]	2.37 [a]	1.77 [b]	2.00 [ab]	1.83 [b]	1.73 [b]
Dusty/Earthy Aroma	2.30 [bc]	2.23 [bc]	2.50 [ab]	2.60 [ab]	2.77 [a]	2.50 [ab]	2.07 [c]	2.43 [abc]
Stale Flavor	2.77 [b]	2.73 [b]	3.03 [ab]	3.07 [ab]	3.00 [ab]	3.23 [a]	2.83 [b]	2.80 [b]
Eggy Flavor	1.10 [a]	1.33 [a]	1.23 [a]	1.17 [a]	0.40 [b]	0.93 [a]	1.40 [a]	1.00 [a]
Bitter Taste	7.57 [b]	6.70 [c]	8.07 [ab]	8.33 [a]	7.93 [ab]	8.30 [a]	7.37 [bc]	7.93 [ab]
Dusty/Earthy Flavor	2.13 [c]	2.23 [c]	2.53 [abc]	2.73 [ab]	2.77 [a]	2.27 [c]	2.33 [bc]	2.43 [abc]
Oxidized Oil Flavor	2.24 [b]	2.23 [b]	2.80 [a]	2.80 [a]	2.20 [b]	2.20 [b]	2.20 [b]	2.23 [b]
Barnyard aftertaste	2.87 [d]	3.17 [bcd]	3.47 [ab]	3.67 [a]	3.43 [ab]	3.00 [cd]	3.20 [bcd]	3.27 [bc]
Stale aftertaste	2.67 [c]	3.00 [ab]	3.10 [ab]	3.17 [a]	2.83 [bc]	3.00 [ab]	2.67 [c]	2.90 [abc]
Bitter aftertaste	8.07 [bcd]	7.93 [cd]	8.70 [ab]	8.90 [a]	8.47 [abcd]	8.63 [ab]	7.87 [d]	8.53 [abc]
Sweet aftertaste	0.20 [ab]	0.03 [bc]	0.00 [c]	0.27 [a]	0.03 [bc]	0.00 [c]	0.13 [abc]	0.00 [c]
Oxidized oil aftertaste	2.20 [b]	2.33 [b]	2.57 [ab]	2.90 [a]	2.33 [b]	2.30 [b]	2.23 [b]	2.27 [b]
Fish aftertaste	1.27 [ab]	1.03 [b]	1.80 [a]	1.80 [a]	1.40 [ab]	1.10 [b]	1.77 [a]	1.27 [ab]
Iron aftertaste	1.77 [c]	2.33 [abc]	2.37 [abc]	2.87 [a]	2.30 [abc]	2.43 [ab]	2.17 [bc]	1.93 [bc]

Appearance attributes porous, grainy, and fibrous were significantly different ($p < 0.05$) among the uncoated treatments (Table 2). The two wheat bran fiber diets, WB1 and WB2, had the highest scores for porous attribute, while the small particle size sugar cane (SC2) has the lowest. Sugar cane large particle size (SC1) had the highest fibrous (more than three point-scales from the second highest score) and grainy appearance level while sugar cane small particle size (SC2) had the lowest level for grainy attribute.

Off-notes oxidized oil and dusty/earthy were significantly different for aroma and flavor among the uncoated treatments. Samples GF6 and GF12 showed the highest oxidized oil aroma and flavor level. Stale, egg, and bitter were significantly different in flavor. Samples GF12 and SC2 were the most bitter while GF3 was the least bitter sample. The samples varied in barnyard, stale, bitter, sweet, oxidized oil, fish, and iron aftertaste. Sample GF12 had the highest bitter aftertaste and was the highest in stale, barnyard, sweet, oxidized oil, and fish aftertaste.

Fracturability, initial crispness, fibrous, and gritty attributes differentiated the uncoated treatments in texture. The largest difference in texture was found in the fibrous attribute. Sample SC1 was more than five points higher than the second highest score among the treatments. For other texture attributes the treatments showed smaller differences.

Least significant differences are shown with superscript letters following the average intensity scores. Letters that are the same for a treatment attribute in a row are not significantly different ($p > 0.05$).

The results indicate that fiber source as well as fiber amount and particle size have an influence on the sensory properties of extruded dog food. For aroma and flavor, the overall differences were not too large across the treatments. Bitter taste and stale and iron aftertaste were examples of flavor attributes that differed among treatments. Sample GF12 (together with sample SC1) showed the highest scores for most of the aftertastes (including off-notes) and the highest bitterness. GF12 had the least particle size and also one of highest levels of total dietary fiber among all treatments, which might be factors contributing to highest intensity scores for various attributes described above. On the other hand, GF3 had the least dietary fiber level, which was probably the reason for its lowest bitter score. Martin *et al.* found that dietary fibers enriched breads were characterized by a higher bitterness together with higher cereal and toasted notes [6]. Sugar cane fibers with large particle size (sample SC1) seemed to influence fibrous texture more than any other type of fibers. Sugar cane samples also showed the lowest fracturability and initial crispness (texture) levels, possibly because the length/size of sugar cane fibers was higher than other fibers, leading to a strengthening effect. This was probably also the reason for the above observation related to fibrous texture and was reflected in appearance as well. SC1 showed the highest scores across the sample set for fibrous and grainy appearance attributes. Treatments with sugar cane fiber (SC1 and SC2) also had the least porous appearance. Interestingly, among all fiber sources, wheat bran appeared to have the least impact on most sensory attributes. WB2 showed lower fracturability and initial crispness than WB1. Smaller particle size has been reported previously to result in lower levels of hardness in the case of extruded cereals [5].

3.1.2. Coated Treatments

The main contributing attributes to aroma of the coated treatments were barnyard, brothy, toasted, grainy, dusty/earthy, cardboard, and hay-like [18]. The main contributing attributes to flavor and taste of these dog foods were barnyard, brothy, toasted, grainy, vitamin, sour, salty, bitter, dusty/earthy, cardboard, and hay-like. The highest intensity was noted for bitter taste (averages 5.94–6.56). Commercial pet foods are typically coated with a palatant; in general, commercial dry dog foods exhibit sensory characteristics such as barnyard, brothy, brown, grain, soy, vitamin, oxidized oil, cardboard, and stale [12]. These attributes were similar to the main flavor and taste attributes detected in experimental dry dog foods in this study.

After coating with poultry fat and a palatant there were few significant differences ($p < 0.05$) found among the treatments (Table 3). Brown and porous appearances were the attributes that varied most among the treatments. Wheat bran treatments WB1 and WB2 were significantly darker brown than sugar cane treatments. The control sample was the lightest brown in appearance. Porous appearance was more apparent for the control and WB2 samples. Toasted aroma was found to be less intense in sample SC2, while dusty/earthy aroma was less intense in sample WB1. Sample WB1 was also less intense in cardboard flavor.

Table 3. Average appearance, aroma, and flavor attribute intensity scores for coated treatments. Significantly different attributes showed only ($p < 0.05$).

Attribute	Treatment				
	CO	**SC1**	**SC2**	**WB1**	**WB2**
Brown Appearance	7.19 [c]	7.69 [ab]	7.50 [bc]	7.94 [a]	7.94 [a]
Porous Appearance	2.44 [a]	1.88 [b]	1.81 [b]	1.25 [c]	2.38 [a]
Toasted Aroma	3.38 [a]	3.00 [a]	2.56 [b]	3.13 [a]	3.19 [a]
Dusty/earthy Aroma	2.94 [a]	2.94 [a]	2.88 [a]	2.44 [b]	3.06 [a]
Cardboard Flavor	3.19 [a]	3.13 [a]	2.81 [a]	2.31 [b]	2.81 [a]

Least significant differences are shown with superscript letters following the average intensity scores. Letters that are the same for a treatment attribute in a row are not significantly different ($p > 0.05$).

3.1.3. Coating Effect on Sensory Properties

Poultry fat and palatant effects on appearance, aroma, and flavor attributes among the uncoated and coated treatments were noticed. The coated treatments were less porous in appearance, albeit more intense in brown color. The aromatics of the treatments changed after coating with the poultry fat and palatant (Figure 1). Specifically, stale, liver, and fish aromatics were present in the uncoated kibbles, but were not detected in the coated kibbles. Similarly, sour aromatics and hay-like aroma was detected only in the coated kibbles. Brothy, grainy, and toasted attributes increased in intensity and oxidized oil and iron aromatics reduced in intensity after coating with poultry fat and palatant. The flavor of the treatments changed after coating with the poultry fat and palatant (Figure 2). Fish flavor was not detected in the coated kibbles, while hay-like flavor was detected in the coated kibbles. Brothy, toasted, and grainy flavor increased after coating the kibbles. Stale, liver, oxidized oil, metallic, and iron flavor and bitter taste decreased after coating the kibbles. It was apparent that coating had a masking effect on appearance attributes such as porosity, aroma attributes such as stale, and flavor attributes such as iron and bitter taste.

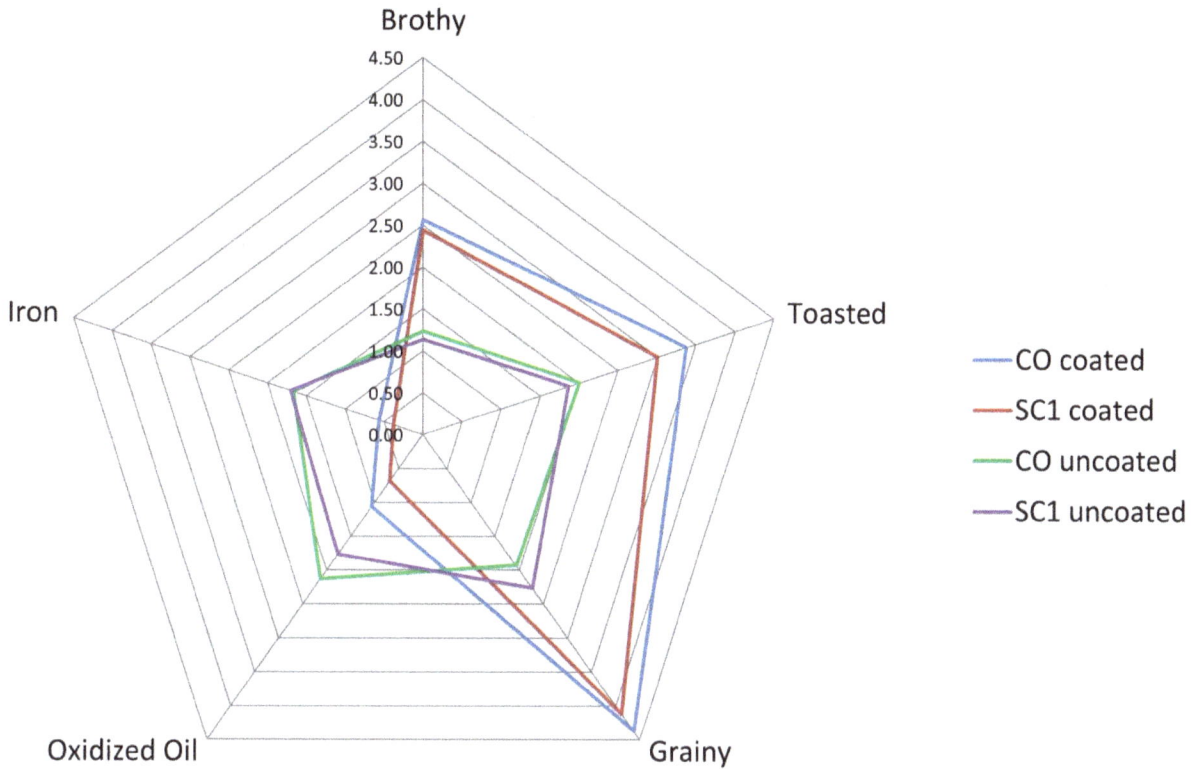

Figure 1. Poultry fat and palatant effect on kibble aromatics. Only the Control (CO) sample and Sugar Cane large particles (SC1) samples are shown.

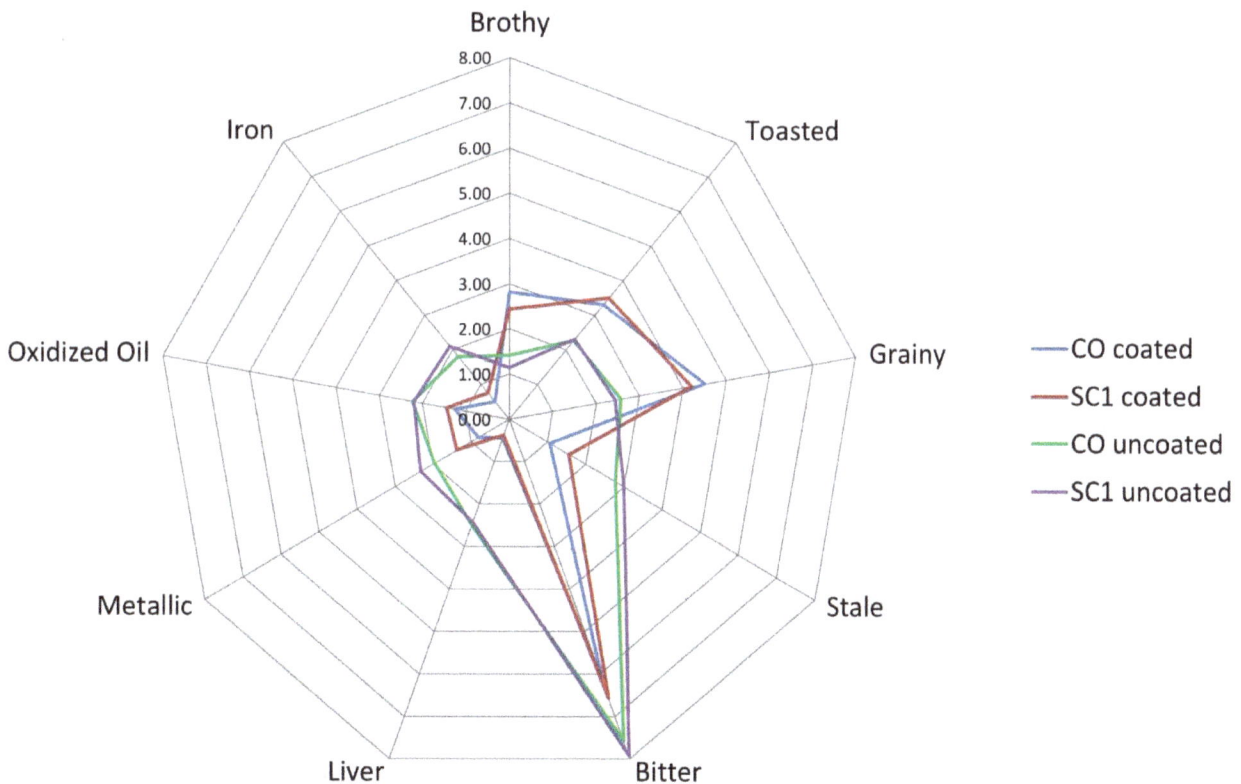

Figure 2. Poultry fat and palatant effect on kibble flavor. Only the Control (CO) sample and Sugar Cane large particles (SC1) samples are shown.

3.2. Palatability

According to the palatability testing results some of the treatments were more palatable than others (Table 4). For example the CO treatment was eaten more than SC2 or WB2, thus implying that fiber addition decreased the palatability. This is not a surprising result, given the negative attributes associated with fiber in general, including hardness and bitterness. A study conducted by Sa *et al.* [10] looked at using wheat bran in dog foods. These authors found that the dogs in the experiment actually consumed the negative control sample less than the wheat bran treatments, however, this was not a preference test. Sample WB1 was eaten more than WB2, and SC1 was eaten more than SC2. These results indicated that both fiber addition and the size of the fiber particles might have an influence when determining whether the diet is palatable or not. A full set of comparisons among the treatments would be needed in order to determine an order of preference.

Table 4. Palatability testing results.

Comparison	Treatment	First Choice (%)	Food intake (%)
CONTROL *versus* SC2	Control	70 **	80 ***
	SC2	30	20
CONTROL *versus* WB2 *	Control	75 **	88 ***
	WB2	25	12
SC1 *versus* SC2	SC1	87 ***	79 ***
	SC2	13	21
WB1 *versus* WB2	WB1	24	55
	WB2	76 **	45

* This test was not validated due to underconsumption of the treatments by the dogs. ** difference between groups ($p < 0.05$). *** difference between groups ($p < 0.01$).

3.3. Potential Effect of Sensory Properties on Palatability

Further inspection of the treatments sensory properties and palatability testing results indicated that the texture properties of CO and WB1 were similar in fracturability, initial crispness, and fibrous attributes. The CO sample was preferred over both SC2 and WB2. The WB1 sample was only compared to WB2 sample, and the results showed a somewhat higher, but not significantly higher intake for WB1 sample (Table 4). These results indicate that texture properties may have an influence on dry pet food palatability, and higher intensity of attributes such as fracturability and initial crispness might lead to greater palatability.

Most variability was detected in the fibrous texture attribute. This was probably caused by the different fiber sources used in the formulation. The CO and WB1 samples were similarly low in this attribute, while WB2 and SC2 were higher, and SC1 the highest (9.20, Table 2). The fibrous attribute was defined as "the perception of fibers and filaments in the product after three to five chews". Most dogs do not chew the food too extensively, but the fibrous texture is likely to have an impact on the mouthfeel of the food. Based on the results from palatability testing, it seems that fibrous mouthfeel may have an effect on pet food preference. When considering that SC1 was preferred over SC2, however, and that SC1 was highest in fibrous characteristics, the role of this attribute in determining palatability should be studied further.

There were only three aroma and flavor attributes that were significantly different among the coated treatments (toasted and dusty/earthy aroma and cardboard flavor). Toasted aromatics were the highest in the CO sample, and lowest in SC2 sample. As the CO was eaten more in the comparisons, and SC2 was eaten less in the comparisons, this attribute may be important in determining palatability of dry pet food. The texture effect was expected to be more prominent in these treatments, as the palatant amount and formulation was kept constant for each of the treatments. Nevertheless these differences in aroma and flavor were likely to be the result of the ingredient differences and may have influenced palatability as well.

In a comparison between WB1 and WB2, WB2 was most often the first choice for dogs. This did not result in this sample being the most eaten, though. Treatment WB2 showed a higher dusty/earthy aromatics level, and this could be a factor that attracted the dogs before they actually started eating. A flavor note that was different between WB1 and WB2 was cardboard, and WB2 had a higher intensity of this flavor. This may be one of the reasons for preference of WB1 once dogs started eating the treatment.

A Principal Components Analysis (PCA) was conducted in order to visualize the main differences between the treatments and to relate these to dog preference testing results. A total of 78.54% of variability among the treatments was explained by the two first Principal Components (Figure 3). According to the PCA analysis in the comparison of treatments WB1 and WB2, porous appearance and cardboard flavor and dusty/earthy aromatics may have influenced palatability. The comparison between CO and WB2 or SC2 resulted in the CO treatment being more palatable. This may have been caused by higher toasted aromatics, grittiness, initial crispness, or fracturability. The comparison between SC1 and SC2 resulted in the SC1 treatment being more palatable. This may have been caused by the more fibrous texture of treatment SC1.

There are some limitations to this research. The first and most obvious is the fact that human senses are different from a dog's senses. This study was not trying to claim that the senses of a human and those of a dog are similar. Rather the study was trying to understand if there were any sensory attributes that the human panelists could distinguish in dog foods that may help indicate direction of preference in a palatability test. While the results from this study may not necessarily fully answer that question, at least as far as fiber sources in pet foods are concerned, some indication of the reasons behind higher liking were detected.

The second limitation lies in the palatability test and the amount of information collected with this test. Typically, characteristics like first choice and food intake are collected. During an eating situation, dogs, just like humans, are likely to indicate their liking with other bodily cues, such as wagging the tail, increased heart rate or respiration rate, pupil dilation, licking of the mouth, or other indications. A study conducted by van den Bos *et al.* [19] concluded that cats might indicate their liking or disliking of foods with some behavioral, facial or tongue movements. Further research is needed to understand what cues may indicate liking in dogs. In addition, the two-bowl testing situations are somewhat forced in their nature. The dogs have two choices of food to choose from, and there is no guarantee that either of the foods is more palatable. Since the dogs are likely to be hungry, they will probably eat either or both of the foods, but this may not necessarily show that either of the foods is liked more.

Biplot (axes F1 and F2: 78.54 %)

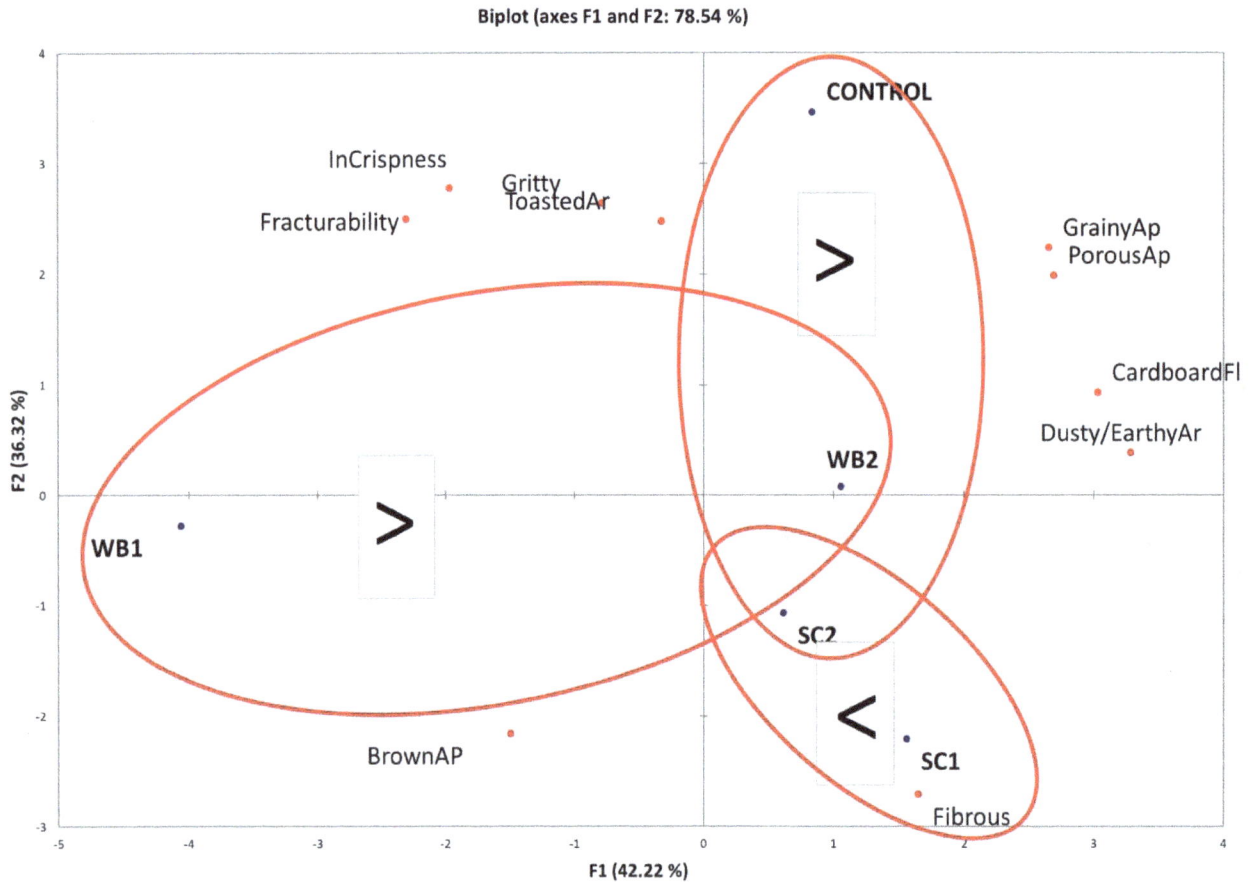

Figure 3. Principal Components Analysis of treatments for the significantly different appearance (Ap) texture, aroma (Ar), and flavor (Fl) attributes. Texture attributes were included based on the uncoated treatment descriptive sensory analysis results. In Crispness—Initial crispness. The < and > symbols indicate the direction of the palatability test for the comparisons of samples within the ovals.

Furthermore, the use of kennel dogs may provide different results than the use of actual pets that live with their owners. This has been shown by Smith et al. [20] in a comparison of laboratory and pet dogs in their preferences for dog foods that varied in flavor. In the current study, the focus was on texture attributes, as the flavor variation was kept at a minimum by using the same palatant on all treatments. A comparison of different textures of dog foods has been conducted by Kitchell et al. [21], however this comparison was among moist, canned, and dry foods. A preference of canned and moist foods over dry foods was found in that study. No studies were found that compared dog preference for different dry food textures.

4. Conclusions

The results of this study indicated that fibers (type or quality, particle size, and amount) have an influence on sensory characteristics of extruded dog food. The texture of treatments was most influenced by the different fibers, and sugar cane fibers with large particle size influenced the fibrousness of treatments more than other fiber sources. Moreover, the higher length of sugar cane fibers, causing a strengthening effect, could have played a role in the lowest score in fracturability and initial crispness. Fibers seemed to influence aroma and flavor properties; the treatment with the highest amount of guava fibers was the most bitter and had most aftertastes, including off-notes such as stale and oxidized oil. The coating process showed to be fundamental in reducing or eliminating off-notes both in flavor and aroma, and also altering the appearance. Moreover it increased notes such as brothy, grainy, and toasted in the samples and even added new characteristics not present in the uncoated samples such as sour taste and hay-like aroma and flavor.

Palatability testing results indicated that the control treatment was preferred over treatments containing small particle size of both sugar cane and wheat bran fibers. Product hardness, bitter taste and other off-notes associated with fibers might have been contributing factors. When the same fiber sources where compared, a preference for large particle size was shown for the food intake. Wheat bran fibers with small particle size showed to be preferred as first choice but not in regard to food intake.

Results showed that texture characteristics such as fracturability, initial crispness, and grittiness, together with aromas such as toasted may play a main role in increasing the palatability. Moreover, different results among first choice and food intake for a particular source of fiber may be helpful to indicate what kind of aromas may be more attractive for dogs, and what kind of flavors may cause them prefer a treatment that was perhaps not chosen in the first moment.

Further future studies on the subject may clarify the influence of different fibers on palatability further and give a better understanding of the relationship between sensory properties of extruded dog food and acceptance by dogs.

Acknowledgments

The authors thank Dilumix (Leme, SP, Brazil) for processing and donating the fiber sources, and for partially financially supporting the experiment, and Panelis (Diana Group, Descalvado, São Paulo, Brazil) for their technical contribution and donation of the palatability tests with dogs. The authors would also like to thank Jeff Wilson from USDA-ARS Grain Marketing and Production Research Center for the particle size analysis.

Author Contributions

Kadri Koppel was responsible for planning the study, conducting sensory analysis, writing and editing the manuscript, and analyzing the sensory data. Mariana Monti was responsible for planning the study, manufacturing the diets, reviewing the manuscript, and analyzing the diets composition. Michael Gibson was responsible for manufacturing the diets, planning the study, and reviewing the manuscript. Sajid Alavi was responsible for planning the study and composing and reviewing the manuscript. Brizio Di Donfrancesco was responsible for conducting the sensory analysis and reviewing the manuscript. Aulus Carciofi was responsible for planning the study, manufacturing the diets, organizing palatability trials, and composing and reviewing the manuscript.

Conflicts of Interest

The authors declare no conflict of interest.

References

1.   Mcnamara, J.P. Chapter 3: Glucose and Fatty Acids: Providers of Body Structure and Function. In *Principles of Companion Animal Nutrition*, 2nd ed.; Pearson Education, Inc.: Upper Saddle River, NJ, USA, 2014; pp. 27–47.

2.   Weber, M.; Bissot, T.; Servet, E.; Sergheraert, R.; Biourge, V.; German, A.J. A high-protein, high-fiber diet designed for weight loss improves satiety in dogs. *J. Vet. Int. Med.* **2007**, *21*, 1203–1208.

3.   De Godoy, M.R.C.; Kerr, K.R.; Fahey, G.C., Jr. Alternative dietary fiber sources in companion animal nutrition. *Nutrients* **2013**, *5*, 3099–3117.

4.   Campbell, K.L.; Campbell, J.R. Chapter 9: Feeding and Nutrition of Dogs and Cats. In *Companion Animals. Their Biology, Care, Health, and Management*, 2nd ed.; Pearson Education Inc.: Upper Saddle River, NJ, USA, 2009; pp. 253–299.

5.   Robin, F.; Schuchmann, P.H.; Palzer, S. Dietary fiber in extruded cereals: Limitations and opportunities. *Trends Food Sci. Tech.* **2012**, *28*, 23–32.

6.   Martin, C.; Chiron, H.; Issanchou, S. Impact of dietary fiber enrichment on the sensory characteristics and acceptance of French baguette. *J. Food Qual.* **2013**, *36*, 324–333.

7.   Wang, J.; Rosell, C.M.; Benedito de Barber, C. Effect of the addition of different fibers on wheat dough performance and bread quality. *Food Chem.* **2002**, *79*, 221–226.

8.   Popov-Ralić, J.V.; Mastilović, J.S.; Laličić,-Petronijević, J.G.; Kevrešan, Z.S.; Demin, M.A. Sensory and color properties of dietary cookies with different fiber sources during 180 days of storage. *Hem. Ind.* **2013**, *67*, 123–134.

9.   Pacheco, G.F.E.; Marcolla, C.S.; Machado, G.S.; Kessler, A.M.; Trevizan, L. Effect of full-fat rice bran on palatability and digestibility of diets supplemented with enzymes in adult dogs. *J. Anim. Sci.* **2014**, *92*, 4598–4606.

10. Sa, F.C.; Vasconcellos, R.S.; Brunetto, M.A.; Filho, F.O.R.; Gomes, M.O.S.; Carciofi, A.C. Enzyme use in kibble diets formulated with wheat bran for dogs: Effects on processing and digestibility. *J. Anim. Physiol. Anim. Nutr.* **2013**, *97*, 51–59.

11. Koppel, K. Sensory analysis of pet foods. *J. Sci. Food Agric.* **2014**, *94*, 2148–2153.

12. Di Donfrancesco, B.; Koppel, K.; Chambers, E., IV. An initial lexicon for sensory properties of dry dog food. *J. Sens. Stud.* **2012**, *27*, 498–510.

13. Koppel, K.; Adhikari, K.; di Donfrancesco, B. Volatile compounds in dry dog foods and their influence on sensory aromatic profile. *Molecules* **2013**, *18*, 2646–2662.

14. Koppel, K.; Gibson, M.; Alavi, S.; Aldrich, G. The effects of cooking process and meat inclusion on pet food flavor and texture characteristics. *Animals* **2014**, *4*, 254–271.

15. FEDIAF—European Pet Food Industry Federation. Nutritional Guidelines for Complete and Complementary Pet Food for Cats and Dogs. 2011. Available online: http://www.fediaf.org/press-area/press-releases/news-detail/artikel/nutritional-guidelines-cats-and-dogs/ (accessed on 26 November 2014).

16. Boac, J.M.; Maghirang, R.G.; Casada, M.E.; Wilson, J.D.; Jung, Y.S. Size distribution and rate of dust generated during grain elevator handling. *Appl. Eng. Agric.* **2009**, *25*, 533–541.

17. Griffin, R.W. Section IV: Palatability. In *Petfood Technology*, 1st ed.; Kvamme, J.L., Phillips, T.D., Eds.; Watt Publishing Co.: Mt Morris, IL, USA, 2003; pp. 176–193.

18. Koppel, K. The Sensory Analysis Center, Department of Human Nutrition, College of Human Ecology, Kansas State University, Manhattan, KS, USA. Unpublished data. 2014.

19. Van den Bos, R.; Meijer, M.K.; Spruijt, B.M. Taste reactivity patterns in domestic cats (*Felis silvestris catus*). *Appl. Anim. Behav. Sci.* **2000**, *69*, 149–168.

20. Smith, S.L.; Kronfeld, D.S.; Banta, C.A. Owners' perception of food flavor preferences of pet dogs in relation to measured preferences of laboratory dogs. *Appl. Anim. Ethol.* **1983**, *10*, 75–87.

21. Kitchell, R.L.; Franti, C.E.; Sprague, R.H. Palatability of commercial dog foods. *Anat. Histol. Embryol.* **1975**, *4*, 371.

9

A Reproductive Management Program for an Urban Population of Eastern Grey Kangaroos (*Macropus giganteus*)

Andrew Tribe [1,5], Jon Hanger [2], Ian J. McDonald [1], Jo Loader [2], Ben J. Nottidge [3], Jeff J. McKee [4] and Clive J. C. Phillips [5,*]

[1] School of Agriculture and Food Sciences, University of Queensland, Gatton, Queensland 4343, Australia; E-Mails: a.tribe@uq.edu.au (A.T.); ianmcd85@hotmail.com (I.J.M.)
[2] Endeavour Veterinary Ecology Pty Ltd, Toorbul, Queensland 4510, Australia; E-Mails: jonhanger@hotmail.com (J.H.); jo@endeavourvet.com.au (J.L.)
[3] GreenLeaf Ecology, Mooloolah, Queensland 4553, Australia; E-Mail: ben@glecology.com.au
[4] Ecosure, West Burleigh, Queensland 4219, Australia; E-Mail: jmckee@ecosure.com.au
[5] Centre for Animal Welfare and Ethics, University of Queensland, Gatton, Queensland 4343, Australia

* Author to whom correspondence should be addressed; E-Mail: c.phillips@uq.edu.au.

Simple Summary: We designed a programme to control free-ranging kangaroos on a Queensland golf course, using contraceptive implants in females and vasectomisation or testicle removal in males. This reduced the numbers of pouch young to about one half of pre-intervention levels and controlled the population over a 2–4 year period. However, the necessary darting caused a mortality rate of 5–10% of captured animals, mainly due to complications before and after anaesthesia. It is concluded that population control is possible but careful management of kangaroos around the time of anaesthesia induction and recovery is important in such programmes to minimise losses.

Abstract: Traditionally, culling has been the expedient, most common, and in many cases, the only tool used to control free-ranging kangaroo populations. We applied a reproductive control program to a population of eastern grey kangaroos confined to a golf course in South East Queensland. The program aimed to reduce fecundity sufficiently for the population to decrease over time so that overgrazing of the fairways and the frequency of human–animal conflict situations were minimised. In 2003, 92% of the female kangaroos above 5 kg bodyweight were implanted with the GnRH agonist deslorelin after darting with a dissociative anaesthetic. In 2007, 86% of the females above 5 kg were implanted with deslorelin and also 87% of the males above 5 kg were sterilised by either orchidectomy or vasectomy. In 2005, 2008 and 2009, the population was censused to assess the effect of each treatment. The 2003 deslorelin program resulted in effective zero population growth for approximately 2.5 years. The combined deslorelin–surgery program in 2007 reduced the birth rate from 0.3 to 0.06%/year for 16 months, resulting in a 27% population reduction by November 2009. The results were consistent with implants conferring contraception to 100% of implanted females for at least 12 months. The iatrogenic mortality rates for each program were 10.5% and 4.9%, respectively, with 50% of all mortalities due to darting-related injuries, exertional myopathy/hyperthermia or recovery misadventure. The short term sexual and agonistic behaviour of the males was assessed for the 2007 program: no significant changes were seen in adult males given the vasectomy procedure, while sexual behaviours' were decreased in adult males given the orchidectomy procedure. It is concluded that female reproduction was effectively controlled by implantation with deslorrelin and male reproductive behaviour was reduced by orchidectomy, which together achieved population control.

Keywords: behaviour; Deslorelin; orchidectomy; vasectomy; welfare

---

1. Introduction

Loss and fragmentation of wildlife habitats and the ecological consequences that follow are major challenges for nature conservation. While loss of biodiversity is one of the most concerning trends, local overabundance, particularly in isolated habitat remnants, may lead to human–animal conflicts and undesirable ecological effects requiring intervention. It is important that management of overabundant species is effective, ecologically sound, humane and socially acceptable.

Since European settlement, the eastern grey kangaroo (*Macropus giganteus*) is one Australian species that is said to have benefited from habitat changes, increasing in population size and range along the eastern coast and for some distance inland [1,2]. Within Australian society, the kangaroo is perceived both as an iconic national symbol and but also invasive in many areas, hence opinion regarding management options varies from full protection to unrestricted culling [3]. However, because of perceived animal welfare and ethical issues and increased availability of non-lethal options, culling is now under greater public scrutiny and socio-political restraint. Non-lethal management options, including translocation and partial or complete reproductive suppression of a population, have greater appeal and hence are the subjects of ongoing investigation [4–8].

Although non-lethal management options may be more socio-politically acceptable, there are nevertheless potential risks to animal welfare associated with capture, anaesthesia and surgical procedures that must be mitigated if such methods are to be widely accepted. Furthermore, behavioural changes associated with pharmacological or surgical intervention may affect the dominance hierarchy and social structure within a population [9–12]. This may reduce group cohesion, which increases their vulnerability in a semi-porous containment area, such as a golf course. Reduced sexual activity may in particular reduce group cohesion.

Herbert *et al.* [5] demonstrated that the gonadotrophin-releasing hormone (GnRH) agonist deslorelin is an effective contraceptive in female eastern grey kangaroos. In their study, the mean contraceptive period for sustained-release implants containing 10 mg of deslorelin was approximately 18 months. Nave *et al.* [8] and Couslon *et al.* [6] demonstrated periods of contraception of approximately 27–48 months in female eastern grey kangaroos after treatment with levonorgestrel implants.

Surgical sterilisation results in permanent reproductive impairment, but is more invasive, labour intensive and requires specialist training. Male vasectomy and distal oviductal transection of females are two methods that have been used to control fecundity in the Kangaroo Island koala population successfully [13]. Castration has not, to our knowledge, been used for suppression of reproduction in wild kangaroo populations, but orchidectomy and vasectomy are routine, safe procedures used for sterilising male captive macropods in zoological collections [14] and to our knowledge have been used in one urban population of kangaroos in Canberra [15]. At present, the behavioural and social effects of a reproductive management program involving a variety of fertility control techniques, such as hormonal contraception and surgical sterilisation, in wild kangaroos have not been documented.

The aim of the reproductive management program reported here was to achieve zero or negative growth in a kangaroo population using a combination of fertility control methods, namely the use of deslorelin implants in females and surgical sterilisation of males using orchidectomy or vasectomy. The mean yearly percentage reduction in recruitment, the effective population growth rates and the cost per percent reduction in recruitment achieved using deslorelin alone are reported and compared with a combination of deslorelin and surgical sterilisation. In addition, the iatrogenic morbidity and mortality rates associated with capture and restraint and the percentage reduction in agonistic and sexual behaviours associated with vasectomy and orchidectomy have been summarised.

2. Methods

2.1. Study Site

This study was conducted on a 100 hectare golf course situated on the Gold Coast, Queensland, Australia (Figure 1). In 2003, the course was bounded on its northern and western sides by high density residential areas, on its eastern side by a marine inlet, and on its southern side by a grassland area under preparation for residential development. Since that time, the adjacent block on the southern side has been developed as a high-density residential precinct. The southern and western boundaries of the golf course were contained by a 2 m high chainmesh fence, porous in places. The course contained a number of artificial freshwater lakes and waterways and large and small "roughs" vegetated by stands of pine (*Pinus spp.*) or mixed native and exotic vegetation.

In 2003, the managers of the golf course were concerned that the current kangaroo population size could increase the risk of human injury and cause damage to fairways and greens from overgrazing. Consequently, they elected to explore management options. Culling was not considered for ethical, public safety and public relations reasons.

Figure 1. Map showing Pines golf course and surrounding urban areas (Google Earth, 2009).

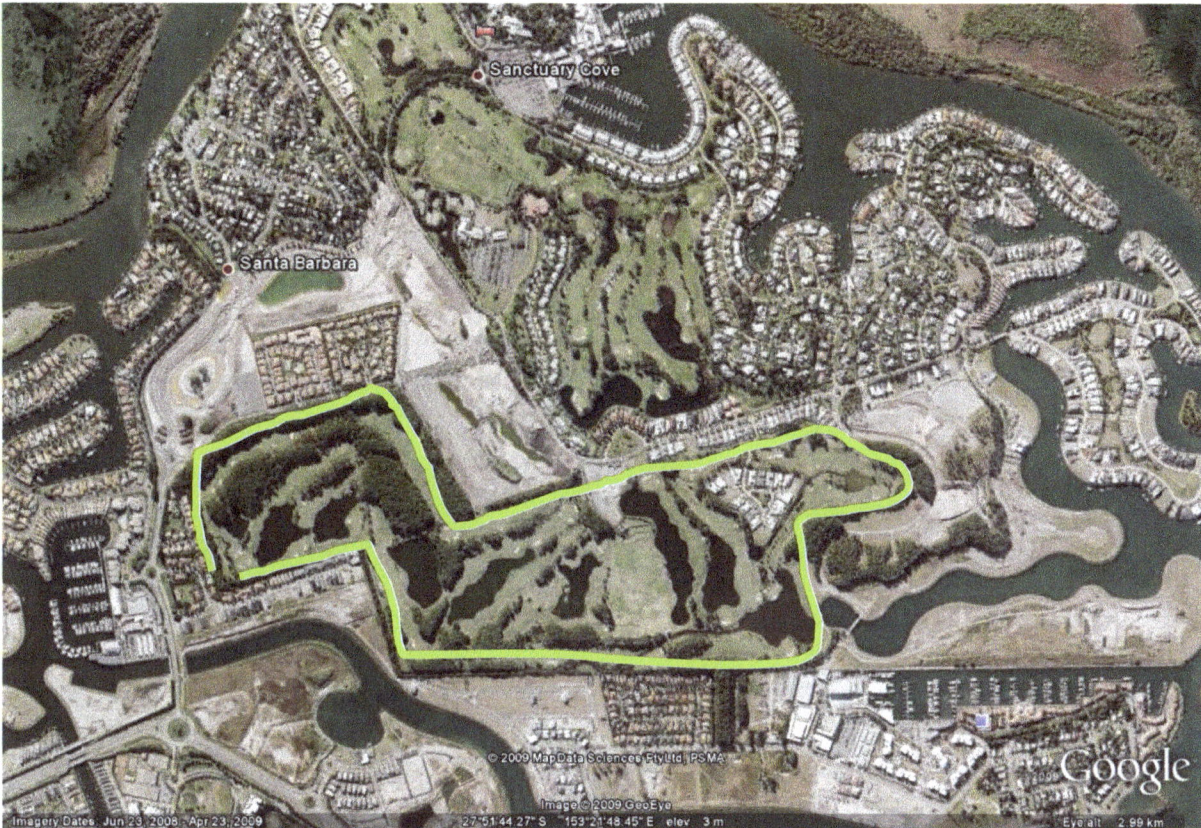

2.2. The Eastern Grey Kangaroo Population

Notwithstanding the issues with fence integrity, the eastern grey kangaroo population was mainly confined to the golf course. The kangaroos followed a typical crepuscular activity pattern, and during the middle of the day rested in variably-sized mobs in some of the roughs. Anecdotally, the causes of premature mortality in the population were motor vehicle strike on adjacent roads and fox predation on young animals. The kangaroos were habituated to the presence of golfers and their buggies. For the purposes of this study, "flight distance" was defined as the minimum human to animal distance at which kangaroos took flight or displayed avoidance behaviour. We observed that for most kangaroos on the golf course flight distances were in the order of 5–10 m, although this distance increased to 10–35 m over the capture period.

2.3. Census

An initial count of the kangaroo population was undertaken in 2003 by Wildcare Population Health Services. The estimated population at the time was believed to be 194 kangaroos. In 2007, two methods were used to count kangaroos and record basic demographic data:

Method 1: All kangaroos were observed with binoculars to determine sex, age group (adult, sub-adult) and presence of pouch young. This method was the slower of the two and increased the likelihood of double counting due to milling.

Method 2: Kangaroos were counted rapidly irrespective of age and sex class and excluded pouch young.

Kangaroo numbers were assessed from a moving buggy, which stopped if the numbers of kangaroos were too many to count instantaneously. Population estimates were based on the number counted by method 2 plus the number of pouch young observed by method 1, multiplied by a correction factor of 1.2 to allow for undetectable pouch young. This correction factor was based on our estimate that approximately one sixth of pouch young were too small to be detected during the census.

2.4. Capture Restraint and Reproductive Control

The first of two reproductive control programs occurred between August and September 2003. As many as possible of the adult and juvenile kangaroos more than 5 kg were captured by projectile anaesthesia, clinically assessed and tagged. Only females weighing more than 5 kg were implanted with deslorelin-containing slow-release implants (Suprelorin 12®, 9.4 mg deslorelin, Peptech Animal Health). Weight was established by experienced wildlife veterinarians after translocation of each animal. A follow-up census was conducted in November 2005.

The second reproductive control program occurred between May and July 2007. All female kangaroos weighing more than 5 kg were implanted with Suprelorin and all adult and sub-adult male kangaroos more than 5 kg were surgically sterilised. Censuses were conducted in November 2008 and November 2009. A summary of the program timeframes is contained in Table 1.

Table 1. Population management program timeframes.

Time	Activity
March 2003	Initial population estimate
August–September 2003	Capture and tag all kangaroos. Suprelorin implantation of females more than 5 kg only
November 2005	Population census
May–July 2007	Capture and tag all kangaroos. Surgical sterilisation of all males more than 5 kg. Suprelorin implantation of all females above 5 kg
March–September 2007	Behavioural observations
November 2008	Population census
November 2009	Population census

During the 2003 program, kangaroos demonstrated increasing flight distances as darting progressed. After 3 days of continuous capture the animals' flight distances were beyond the safe range of the dart gun and the program was deferred for 2–3 weeks to allow the kangaroos to settle. Thereafter, each capture session occurred over only 2 days with breaks of 2–3 weeks between sessions. The 2003 program was completed in 5 capture days over a total elapsed time of 2 months. The 2007 program was completed in 6 capture days over a total elapsed time of 2 months.

2.5. Kangaroo Capture and Veterinary Procedures

2.5.1. Capture and Anaesthesia

Kangaroos were captured by projectile anaesthesia using Tel-Inject or Dan-Inject re-useable darts fired from either a Taipan 2000 (Montech Industries) or JM Special 25 (Dan-Inject) dart rifle. The anaesthetic agent was Zoletil (tiletamine + zolazepam) (Virbac (Australia), NSW, Australia) delivered at 5–15 mg/kg body weight over darting distances of 5–35 m. Surgeries were performed using standard techniques in a temporary facility observing aseptic techniques. Additional anaesthetic was administered if required. Two darting teams were in operation, consisting of one veterinarian, one veterinary nurse, and one field biologist (spotter), along with kangaroo transport teams consisting of three groups of two wildlife carers which followed each darted kangaroo in a buggy until it was fully immobilised and therefore safe to move. Darting teams returned to the central management area to check on progress with each animal. A veterinary procedures team, consisting of one veterinarian, two veterinary nurses and three volunteer wildlife carers assisted with animal handling and general duties. On arrival, the kangaroo was weighed and placed on the surgery table for a full physical examination and prepared for surgery. A data sheet was then commenced and accompanied the animal to the veterinary procedures area in the golf cart, taking up to 5 minutes.

In 2003, all darted kangaroos were tagged with swivel-type plastic numbered ear tags (Swing-free Tags, Stockbrands, WA, Australia) and marked with temporary stock marking paint to prevent accidental re-darting. Prior to surgery, each kangaroo was given a physical examination to check body condition and gross evidence of any injury or illness, and a cloacal temperature measurement was taken every 15 minutes. Each captured kangaroo was given an injection of Vitamin E + selenium (Ilium Selvite E, Troy Laboratories, Smithfield, NSW, Australia) at a dose rate of 1 mL/30 kg to assist in the prevention of exertional myopathy [16].

All females over 5 kg were injected in the interscapular subcutis with a single 10 mg deslorelin implant (Suprelorin) (Table 2). The following procedures were undertaken on the females:

- checked for pouch young (PY) and if found, the joeys were then sexed and weighed,
- patch of hair shaved and cleaned above the shoulders at the site for the hormonal implant,
- numbered red ear tag placed in the right ear and a red arm band on the right arm.

The following procedures were undertaken on all the males:

- intravenous injection of Alfaxan® to provide a deeper and more stable level of anaesthesia during surgery. Alfaxan® was also useful because of its shorter period of action than Zoletil® particularly when given intravenously,
- scrotum was shaved, cleaned and prepared for surgery,
- castrated males were also given an injection of lignocaine directly into the testes as a local anaesthetic,
- one numbered red ear tag was placed in their left ear,
- one numbered blue ear tag was placed in the right ear and blue arm band was placed on the right arm if the animal was being castrated,
- alternatively, one numbered green ear tag was placed in the right ear and a blue arm band on the left arm if the animal was being vasectomised,
- injection of engemycin, benacillin antibiotics to help prevent post-operative infection and an injection of metacam for additional for pain relief and a consequently less stressful recovery.

Table 2. Summary of census and veterinary procedure data.

Demographic	Procedure	Number of Kangaroos	
		2003 Program	2007 Program
All kangaroos (incl. pouch young)	Estimated number present at time of management intervention [1]	194	286
All kangaroos	Kangaroos darted	124	187
Females > 5 kg	Deslorelin implant	80	107
Males > 50 kg	Vasectomy	0	19
Males < 50 kg	Vasectomy	0	7
Males > 50 kg	Orchidectomy	0	5
Males > 5 and < 50 kg	Orchidectomy	0	52

[1] Includes pouch young that were captured but not treated.

2.5.2. Processing

Male kangaroos over 5 kg bodyweight were surgically sterilised. Most male kangaroos over 50 kg bodyweight were vasectomised to avoid hormonal changes in dominant males, and most males under 50 kg bodyweight were castrated. In addition, for the purposes of comparison, seven sub-adult males <50 kg were vasectomised and five adult males >50 kg were castrated to determine whether any changes in behaviour could be observed which might be attributed to the sterilisation method for the two classes (sub adult and adult) over the period of this study.

Surgical cases or animals with significant dart wounds were injected with an intramuscular dose of Benacillin (Troy Laboratories, Smithfield, NSW, Australia) at a rate of 1 mL per 10 kg of bodyweight and an intramuscular dose of Engemycin (Intervet Australia, Bendigo, Victoria, Australia) at a dose rate of 10 mg/kg of the active component (oxytetracyline 100 mg/mL). Age, sex, weight, ear tag numbers, anaesthetic details, clinical assessment and procedures were recorded for each animal. When the surgery was completed, each animal was carried to the recovery area and allowed to revive from the anaesthetic. At this stage, the data sheet was given to the veterinary nurse at the shaded recovery area to complete as the animal moved into sternal recumbency and finally left the recovery area of its own accord. During the recovery phase, the animal was spray painted carefully on its back with non-toxic paint, colour coded to indicate the processing session. This was done to further identify which kangaroo had already been sterilised or implanted, to facilitate their behavioural data collection and prevent them from being recaptured during the next day or session.

2.6. Behavioural Observations

Behavioural observations were conducted for 6 weeks prior to the start of the 2007 program, for 8 weeks spanning the capture sessions, and for 6 weeks afterwards. Observations were made on two days each week with the aid of binoculars from a golf cart and occurred over 1 hour sessions: once at sunrise (0700–0800), and once just before sunset (1600–1700).

Preliminary observations identified the relevant behaviours to be recorded, using social and agonistic behaviours previously described [17,18]. Sexual behaviours observed in males were 'following and sniffing females' and penis erection, and agonistic behaviours were fighting with other males, chest beating (male kangaroos beating chest repeatedly with fore paws), high walking and grunting noises. These were recorded each time they were performed by either the focal kangaroo or kangaroos within a group, and had to occur for at least 5 seconds to be recorded. Two bouts were recorded if there was a break of 15 or more seconds between behaviours.

Two observational techniques were used to detect behaviours:

(a) Focal animal sampling: one adult and one sub-adult male kangaroo were chosen at random during each observation session. While it would have been preferable to observe the same target kangaroos over the whole period of the study, this was not possible due to the difficulty in locating and identifying particular individuals across the 100 hectare site.

(b) Continuous sampling: the mean frequencies of agonistic and sexual behaviours for all visible sub-adult and adult male and all mature female kangaroos in a mob were recorded. Mobs of at least 15 kangaroos were chosen for behavioural observations to increase the detection of interactive behaviours.

Observations of the kangaroos' reactions to darting were recorded during capture sessions for administration of reproductive control measures. A "darting reaction score" of 1–4 was recorded for each kangaroo darting event (1: kangaroo showed a minimal reaction to the dart with no flight response; 2: kangaroo jumped at the time of impact, and/or showed ongoing irritation or annoyance to the presence of the dart; 3: the kangaroo demonstrated an immediate flight response; 4: the kangaroo demonstrated rapid or immediate collapse or bone fracture).

2.7. Statistical Analysis of Behavioural Observations

The rates of sexual and agonistic behaviour before, during and after the program were compared in both the focal and continuous sampling groups using a chi-squared analysis, including a Bonferroni adjustment for multiple comparisons. The 'following and sniffing females' sexual behaviour observed in adult males during the continuous sampling was analysed using a Kruskal-Wallis test. Both tests were analysed with the Minitab™ statistical analysis program.

3. Results

3.1. Reproduction and Demographic Effects

In early 2003, prior to any active population management, there were approximately 130 kangaroos present on the golf course, not including pouch young. Figure 2(a) shows estimates of projected population growth based on a birth rate of 0.3 of total population with two different mortality rates. This model assumes resources are not limiting and there is no immigration or emigration. Recruitment (birth rate) of 0.3 was based on the number of pouch young present as a proportion of the total kangaroo population at the time of the first management program and was based on an approximate pouch life of joeys of 12 months.

Figure 2(b) shows predicted population growth with annual mortality rates of 10% and 20% for different implant responses; assuming the implant was effective in either all or 50% of animals for 12 months.

In 2003, during the first control program there were approximately 194 kangaroos present, including pouch young, of which 181 (93%) were captured (Table 3). In November 2005, 26 months after the completion of the 2003 program, the estimated kangaroo population including pouch young was 174, including 37 pouch young, suggesting that the population growth was effectively zero over that period. This data is consistent with either of the two middle curves in Figure 2(b): 20% mortality and 50% implant efficacy, or 10% mortality with 100% implant efficacy. At the time of the second program in mid-2007, the population had grown to 286, of which 79 were pouch young (Table 4). This data is most consistent with the curve in Figure 2 representing 10% mortality with 100% implant efficacy.

Figure 2. (**a**) Predicted kangaroo population growth with no intervention; (**b**) Predicted kangaroo population growth with intervention. M is annual mortality rate.

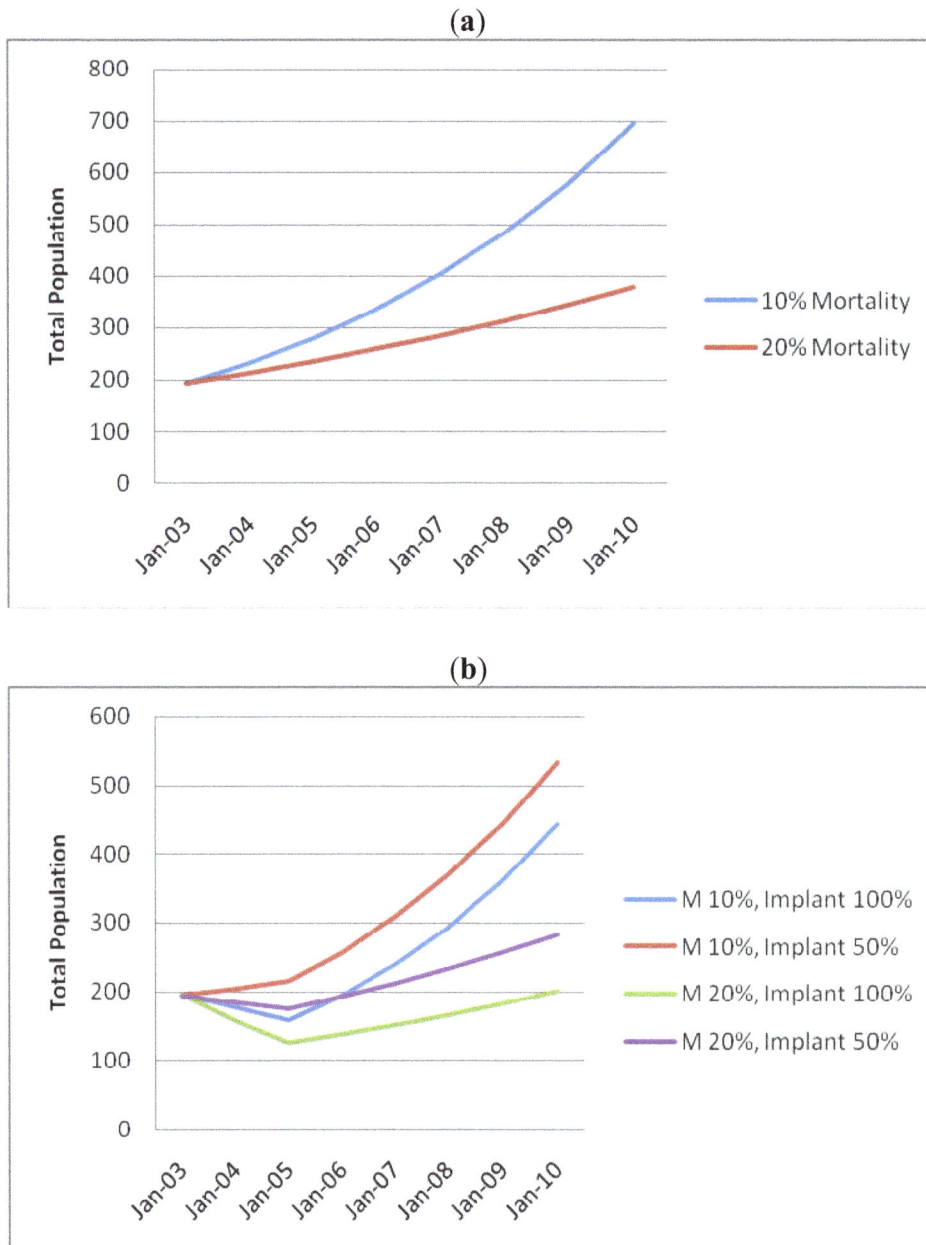

Table 3. Demographic and management data for the 2003 program.

	Above 5 kg		Pouch young	TOTAL
	Males	Females	Unspecified	
Estimated animals present	47	87	60	**194 (100%)**
Total captured	44	80	57	**181 (93%)**
Estimated not captured	3	7	3	**13 (7%)**
Females implanted with deslorelin	-	80	-	**80 (92% of all females)**
Females with pouch young	-	60	-	**60**

Table 4. Demographic and management data for 2007 management intervention.

	Above 5 kg		Pouch Young	Total
	Males	Females	Unspecified	
Estimated animal present	82	125	79	**286 (100%)**
Total captured	72	115	79	**266 (93%)**
Estimated not captured	10	10	0	**20 (7%)**
Male orchidectomy	53	-	-	**53**
Males vasectomy	19	-	-	**19**
Females implanted with deslorelin	-	107	-	**107**
Females with pouch young	-	79	-	**79**
Mortality	11		2	**13**
Number with 2003 tags	40			**40**

Figure 3. Graphical representation of changes in the total number of kangaroos, the number of pouch young and the number of kangaroos excluding pouch young (PY). The timing of management programs is indicated by arrows.

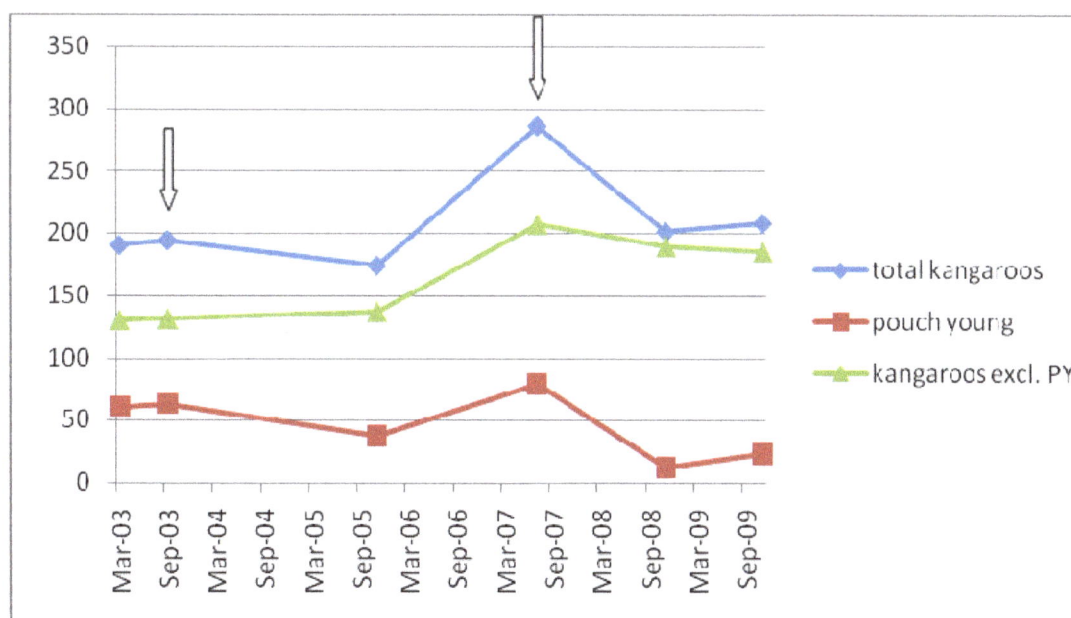

By late 2008, the population had declined to 201, with 12 pouch young and was only marginally greater in November 2009. The estimated number of pouch young decreased from 63 in 2003 to 37 in 2005 then increased to 79 in 2007, finally decreasing to 12 in November 2008. One year later, there were an estimated 23 pouch young, based on the 19 actually observed during the census.

These changes in total kangaroo population and observed pouch young are shown in Figure 3.

The data is consistent with deslorelin implantation of female kangaroos causing a reduction in the average birth rate from 0.3, expressed as a proportion of total population, including pouch young, to close to zero by one year, and a return to 0.2 by 18 months. In comparison, the deslorelin implantation of females plus surgical sterilisation of males caused a more prolonged reduction in birth rate from 0.3 to 0.06 at 16 months and 0.1 at 28 months. The data is confounded to an extent by some immigration to, and emigration from the golf course of up to 20% of the population per year, based on observation of tagged *versus* untagged animals at the censuses [19]).

3.2. Behaviour

3.2.1. Agonistic Behaviours in Males

Agonistic behaviours tended to decrease post-treatment in castrated sub-adult males (<50 kg males) and were not seen at all in the vasectomised sub-adult males (P = 0.001) (Table 5a). Grunting was observed in untreated but not vasectomised or castrated sub-adult males. Grunting behaviour tended to decrease in castrated adult males compared to untreated and vasectomised adult males (P = 0.06). Fighting behaviour was reduced by vasectomisation and castration in sub-adults but not adults (Table 5b).

Table 5. (**a**) Agonistic behaviours in sub-adult and adult male kangaroos during focal and scanning animal sampling observations (analysed by Chi square test); (**b**) Occurrence of fighting behaviour seen in sub-adult and adult male kangaroos during continuous sampling observation sessions; (**c**) Sexually-related behaviours in sub-adult and adult male kangaroos during focal animal sampling observation sessions (analysed by Chi square test).

(**a**) Agonistic behaviour

Age Group	Behaviour		Treatment			P Value		
			U*	V*	O*	U* *vs.* O*	U* *vs.* V*	O* *vs.* V*
Sub-adults	Fighting	Present	10	0	3	0.08	0.001	0.20
		Absent	18	29	25			
	Grunting	Present	8	0	0	0.007	0.006	N/A
		Absent	20	29	28			
Adults	Fighting	Present	5	8	2	0.68	0.76	0.21
		Absent	23	21	22			
	High walking	Present	5	4	1	0.33	0.97	0.55
		Absent	23	25	23			
	Chest beating	Present	3	6	1	0.76	0.66	0.21
		Absent	25	23	23			
	Grunting	Present	8	7	1	0.06	0.97	0.12
		Absent	20	22	23			

U*: Untreated, V*: Vasectomy, O*: Orchidectomy

Table 5. *Cont.*

(**b**) Fighting behaviour

Age Group		Treatment			P Value		
		U*	V*	O*	U* *vs.* O*	U* *vs.* V*	O* *vs.* V*
Sub-adults	Present	6	0	0	0.01	0.01	0.99
	Absent	4	10	10			
Adults	Present	4	2	1	0.32	0.69	0.90
	Absent	6	8	9			

U*: Untreated, V*: Vasectomy, O*: Orchidectomy

(**c**) Sexually-related behaviour

Age Group	Behaviour		Treatment			P Value		
			U*	V*	O*	U* *vs.* O*	U* *vs.* V*	O* *vs.* V*
Sub-adults	Following & sniffing	Present	8	0	1	0.03	0.006	0.664
		Absent	20	29	27			
	Erection	Present	10	0	1	0.007	0.001	0.68
		Absent	18	28	27			
Adults	Following & sniffing	Present	26	21	6	<0.001	0.122	0.002
		Absent	2	8	18			
	Erection	Present	18	19	4	0.002	0.99	0.001
		Absent	10	10	20			

U*: Untreated, V*: Vasectomy, O*: Orchidectomy

3.2.2. Sexual Behaviours in Males

Both castrated and vasectomised sub-adult males had a reduced 'following and sniffing females' behaviour and had fewer erections of the penis compared to the untreated sub-adult males, but in the adult males this was only evident for the castrated and not the vasectomised animals (Table 5c). There was no 'following and sniffing females' behaviour observed in castrated adult male kangaroos, whereas there were 4.5 and 4.0 occurrences observed per hour for the vasectomised and untreated males, respectively ($P < 0.001$, Kruskal-Wallis test) during the continuous sampling.

3.2.3. Female Behaviour

Females that had been implanted spent longer in locomotory behaviour than those that had not (implanted 1.75 *vs.* unimplanted 1.35 $\log_n$ bouts/hour, SED 0.06, $P = 0.04$) and less time scanning (implanted 1.70 *vs.* unimplanted 2.85 $\log_n$ bouts/hour, SED 0.03, $P < 0.001$) and had fewer grooming bouts (implanted 2 *vs.* unimplanted 5 median bouts/hour, $P < 0.001$). There were no significant ($P < 0.05$) differences in feeding, standing or lying behaviour.

3.2.4. Animal Welfare Impact of Management Interventions

3.2.4.1. Response to Darting

Individual responses of kangaroos to darting were recorded only in 2007. Of 187 kangaroos darted, 152 (81%) were given a "darting reaction score". Most females received a score 1 or 2 and most males received a score 2 or 3 (Figure 4). Of the five kangaroos with the maximum darting reaction score of 4, four kangaroos (3%) collapsed immediately, presumably due to deposition of the anaesthetic agent directly into a vein or bone marrow, and one kangaroo suffered a fracture to the tibia, requiring euthanasia.

Figure 4. The kangaroos' immediate physical reactions to being darted during the reproductive management interventions, 2007. 1: kangaroo showed a minimal reaction to the dart with no flight response; 2: kangaroo jumped at the time of impact, and/or showed ongoing irritation or annoyance to the presence of the dart; 3: the kangaroo demonstrated an immediate flight response; 4: the kangaroo demonstrated rapid or immediate collapse or bone fracture.

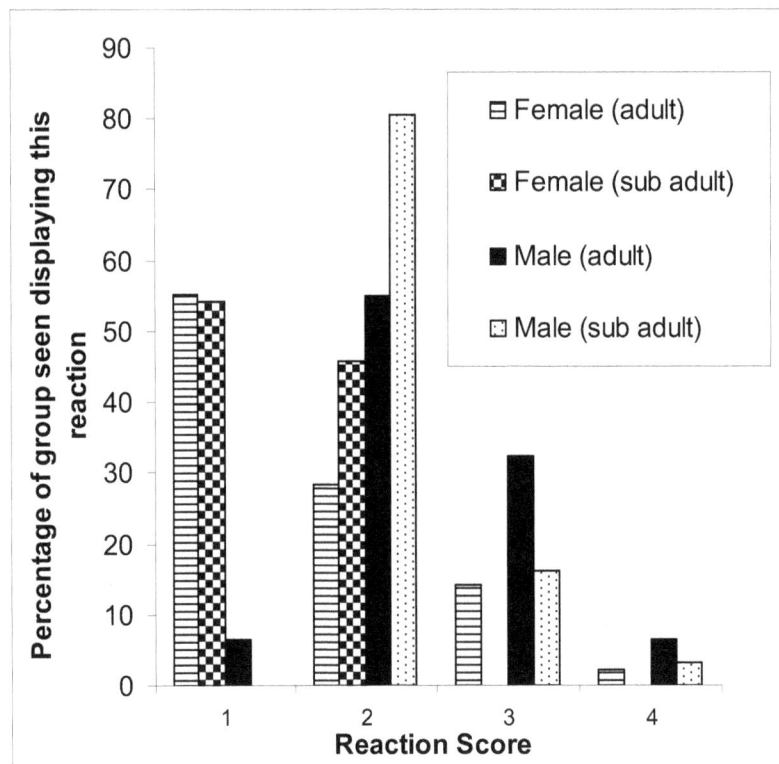

3.2.4.2. Mortality

During both programs, there were darting or anaesthetic mortalities or incidents that required euthanasia. A summary of capture-associated mortalities is presented in Table 6. The animal capture rate (darted animals plus pouch young captured) for both projects was the same (93% of total estimated population), whereas the total mortality rate (as a % of total estimated population) during the 2007 project was less than one half (4.5%) that of the 2003 project (9.8%). Expressed as a percentage of animals captured, the respective mortality rates for 2003 and 2007 were 10.5% and 4.9%.

Five deaths that occurred during recovery from anaesthesia in 2003 were attributed to hyperthermia/myopathy primarily due to high ambient temperatures (26°C or greater). Four animals were found dead up to 2 days after processing and the cause of death was investigated but unclear. Dart-related injuries included fracture of the femur, one spinal injury that required euthanasia and one pouch young that was struck by a dart and died.

In the 2007 management intervention, two kangaroos died as a result of injuries caused by collision with trees during anaesthetic induction after darting. There were three drowning deaths or near-drowning incidents requiring euthanasia that occurred from anaesthesia when kangaroos were ambulatory, but still ataxic.

Table 6. Summary of capture-associated mortalities from the 2003 and 2007 reproductive management plans.

Cause of death/reason for euthanasia	2003 (19 mortalities)		2007 (13 mortalities)		% of all deaths
	Died	Euthanased	Died	Euthanased	
Dart-related injury/fracture	0	5	0	1	19%
Trauma occurring during anaesthetic induction	0	0	0	2	6%
Hyperthermia/myopathy	5	0	1	0	19%
Death after anaesthetic recovery (unspecified cause)	4	0	3	0	22%
Anaesthetic death	0	0	1	0	3%
Drowning/near drowning	0	0	1	2	9%
Predation	2	0	0	0	6%
Untreatable disease	0	1	0	0	3%
Joey death (unviable orphan)	2	0	1	1	13%
Totals	13	6	7	6	100%

3.2.4.3. Non-Lethal Injuries

Non-lethal injuries were generally limited to mild bleeding or haematoma formation at the dart wound requiring minimal veterinary treatment. Virtually all kangaroos experienced a prolonged recovery from anaesthesia (up to 4 hours), during which time they demonstrated significant ataxia and were observed to stand and collapse multiple times, before regaining full coordination and strength.

Spearman's rank correlation indicated a significant positive correlation between the dose rate and the time taken for a full recovery and release from the recovery area back onto the golf course. On average, mature females and males took 154 and 167 minutes, respectively, and sub-adult females and males took 182 and 177 minutes, respectively, to show a full recovery.

In both the 2003 and 2007 management programs, one pouch joey was inadvertently struck by a dart, became anaesthetised and was ejected from the mother's pouch. In 2007, two pouch joeys were abandoned by their mothers during recovery from anaesthesia. All of these joeys were transferred to wildlife carers for hand-rearing and were successfully rehabilitated.

3.2.4.4. Financial Costs and Resource Effort

Each program required 15–20 personnel, including veterinarians, veterinary nurses and wildlife carers. As described in the Method, personnel were divided into three teams: the darting team, consisting of one veterinarian, one veterinary nurse, and one field biologist; the kangaroo transport teams consisting of three groups of two wildlife carers; and the veterinary procedures team, consisting of one veterinarian, two veterinary nurses and three wildlife carers. Additional volunteers (wildlife carers) assisted with animal handling and general duties. The total cost of the 2003 program was AU$18,900, and the 2007 program was AU$49,009.

4. Discussion

4.1. Efficacy of Population Management Program

Based on our population censuses after each program, the reproductive control measures resulted in acceptable reduction of population fecundity, and therefore population growth. Although the census of November 2005 indicated a similar number of adults and sub-adult kangaroos present as were present prior to the 2003 management intervention, the number of pouch young was approximately one half. This result was consistent with our prediction of population number, based upon 100% efficacy of implants and approximately 15% natural attrition (deaths or emigration). At the time of the second management intervention, in mid-2007, the population had increased markedly, with an estimated 207 kangaroos (adults and sub-adults) present, plus approximately 79 pouch young. This is consistent with the expected return of normal fecundity following the loss of effect of the deslorelin implants, as estimated by Herbert and co-workers [5] to be approximately 18 months. However, a significant confounding factor was the potential for movement of kangaroos to and from the site due to numerous breaches in the perimeter fence. At the time of the 2003 management intervention and up to the November 2005 census, there was still a significant population of kangaroos inhabiting or using remnant grassland outside of the golf course, and ample anecdotal evidence of frequent use of breaches in the fence by kangaroos by the course staff and residents. Only 40 of 187 kangaroos darted during the 2007 management intervention had ear tags present from the 2003 management intervention, indicating that a significant proportion of the mature kangaroos present in 2007 were not processed in 2003, and therefore may have immigrated to the site since. In addition, a significant number (estimated to be 20 or more) of kangaroos with ear tags had been killed by motor vehicle strike on roads adjacent to the golf course over the intervening years. By comparison, only 18 of 95 adult kangaroos counted in the November 2008 census were untagged. Given that approximately 20 kangaroos were not captured in the mid-2007 management intervention, the figures are consistent with minimal immigration to the site over that time. Furthermore, urban development had almost entirely destroyed any remnant habitat for kangaroos outside of the golf course by mid-2007.

Our data suggest that deslorelin treatment of female kangaroos alone is sufficient to offer a temporary solution to population growth in eastern grey kangaroos. However, repeat treatments may be required every two years or so, depending upon rates of natural attrition. The addition of surgical (and therefore permanent) sterilisation procedures in male kangaroos was intended to increase the duration of reproductive suppression within the population beyond that provided by deslorelin implantation (of females) alone. Return of fecundity would then rely on the sexual maturation of untreated males (pouch young at the time of the 2007 management intervention), as well as loss of effect of implants in females. In a closed population, this combination is expected to result in a significant drop in the total kangaroo population, followed by a slow increase as normal fecundity returns. However, it is likely that the presence of even a few intact sexually mature males will obviate the effect of permanent sterilisation of other males, as females return to normal reproductive function. The use of levonorgestrel implants in female kangaroos is reported to give a longer period of reproductive suppression compared with deslorelin [6]. Currently, these implants are significantly more expensive than deslorelin implants (AU$250 vs. 60/implant), a factor which will influence cost/% reduction in fecundity/annum. Surgical sterilisation of females, such as by tubal ligation/transection or ovario-hysterectomy, is more invasive than in males and was not considered for financial, ethical and logistic reasons in this program. However, it does offer permanent reproductive control, and is worthy of consideration if financial considerations and other disadvantages are able to be addressed or mitigated. The current programs cost approximately AU$500/year/% reduction in birthrate for GnRH program alone and AU$1050/year/% reduction in birth rate for the deslorelin plus surgery program.

4.2. Animal Welfare Considerations

Anaesthesia and darting of wild animals invariably carry some risk [17]. These risks are associated with:

(1) Injury caused by the dart

(2) Injury or misadventure that occurs during induction or recovery from anaesthesia

(3) Anaesthesia and other veterinary procedures

(4) Predation as a result of impairment of appropriate flight or defence responses [18]

In our program, the mortality rate associated with dart injuries was significantly lower in the second management intervention (8% of all deaths in 2007) than in the first (25% of all deaths in 2003). With respect to the total number of animals actually darted, the figures are 0.5% (2007) and 4% (2003). This difference we attribute primarily to the greater accuracy and finer pressure adjustments of the Dan-Inject dart gun compared with the Montech Taipan 2000. In this program, the target kangaroos were used to human presence, their flight distances were short, and therefore darting distances were significantly shorter than could be expected of kangaroos that were not familiar with humans. This factor contributed significantly to the safety and efficiency of darting capture. We suspected an upward drift in flight distance over time. This could be due to the animals that were easier to dart being targeted first. Alternatively, it could arise from a learnt response to the stress of the darting events. Regular excursions to the site with simulated dart firing prior to a darting event would be one possibility to potentially reduce fear responses.

Injury and mortality associated with anaesthetic induction and recovery were significant. Rapid induction of anaesthesia with minimal excitement is desirable as it reduces the risk of injury and misadventure during the period between darting and recumbency and reduces the likelihood of an animal becoming lost when, or if, it takes flight in response to darting. An accurate weight estimate is essential to calibrate the dose. Tiletamine/zolazepam (Zoletil®, Virbac (Australia), NSW) is a preferred anaesthetic agent for darting of kangaroos because of its short average induction time [17,20,21]. However, it has some significant disadvantages, mainly associated with its prolonged and sometimes violent recovery phase. In addition, in our experience, the risk of serious or fatal hyperthermia in kangaroos anaesthetised with Zoletil is significant at ambient temperatures above approximately 24 °C, because of factors such as tachypnoea and exertion or muscular activity during induction and recovery. We therefore recommend that darting of wild kangaroos not be performed when ambient temperatures are expected to exceed 24 °C at any time between anaesthetic induction and complete recovery. Another factor contributing to poor animal welfare outcomes, and sometimes death of kangaroos, was physical injury that occurred during anaesthetic induction and recovery. Those occurring during anaesthetic recovery may be minimised by confining recovering kangaroos to hessian or shade cloth pens supported at each corner by posts protected by polystyrene padding. These provided some support if the kangaroo knocked into the sides during recovery, whilst minimising injuries. We also avoided excessive disturbance or noise during this phase and used removable eye masks to decrease the amount of light when kangaroos were recovering. Avoiding injuries during anaesthetic induction is somewhat more difficult, but may be minimised by a quiet and calm approach to darting, and avoiding disturbance of chasing darted kangaroos during the induction phase of anaesthesia. Various anaesthetic combinations, including the use of the reversible agents medetomidine and xylazine, were tried in our program, but resulted in unacceptably longer and less predictable anaesthetic induction times when used at recommended dose rates [16]. Consequently, we used Zoletil as our primary agent, despite the issues associated with recovery from anaesthetic [22,23]. In our study, recovery time was longer following higher anaesthetic dose rates (Figure 5). Further development of safe and rapid-induction anaesthetic regimes with superior recovery characteristics to Zoletil may significantly reduce morbidity and mortality associated with anaesthetic recovery. Other important considerationsrelatedto high-volume macropod anaesthesia include human safety issues, costs (of anaesthetic drugs and reversal agents) and the limitations of dart volume.

Figure 5. Time taken to full recovery* from anaesthetic (Zoletil$^®$) during the 2007 intervention at the Pines golf course.

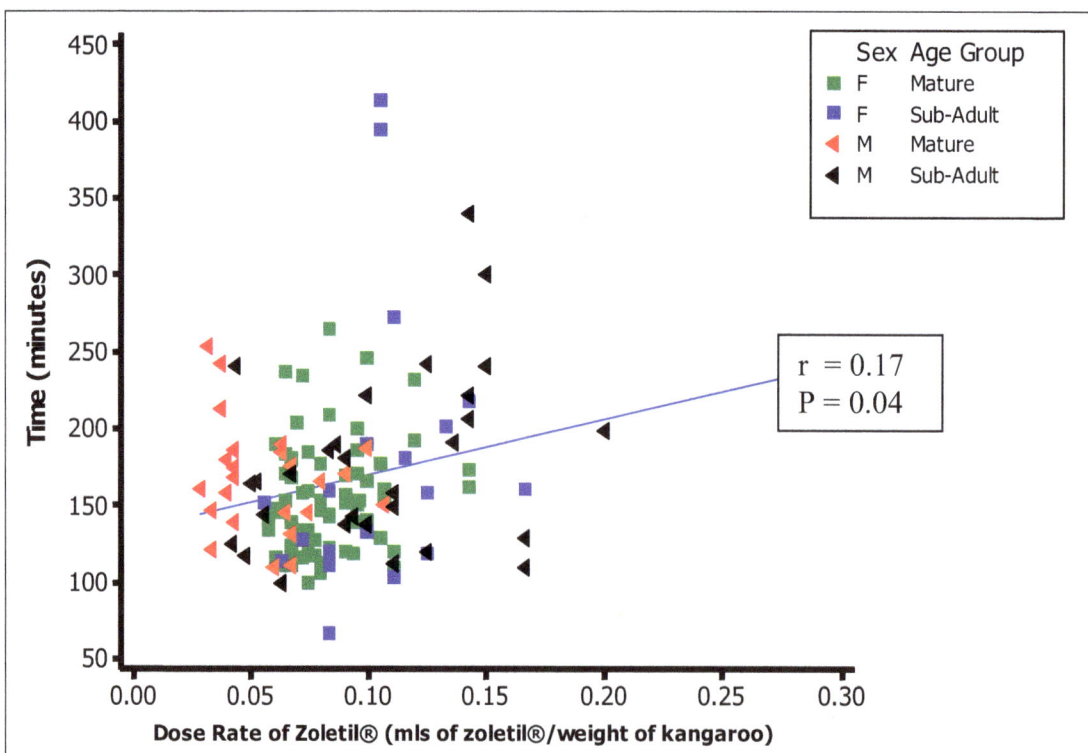

* Kangaroo was able to maintain balance and move away from the recovery area of its own accord.

4.2.1. Animal Reaction to Darting

Most kangaroos displayed only a minimal reaction to the impact of the dart, suggesting that darting generally did not inflict significant pain. As this program involved a population of kangaroos highly habituated to close human presence, it is possible that different reactions would be observed if kangaroos were not as habituated to humans or vehicles. The most serious welfare impacts associated with darting and anaesthesia were those associated with recovery from anaesthesia, during which time kangaroos were prone to injury and hyperthermia, which in some instances led to death.

4.2.2. Short Term Behavioural Responses of Kangaroos to Reproductive Procedures

The results demonstrate that some agonistic behaviours, such as fighting and grunting, still occurred in the sub-adult male kangaroos given the orchidectomy procedure 6–8 weeks post surgery. However, compared with the males given the vasectomy procedure and with observations of untreated sub-adult males during the pre-treatment period, the frequency of these behaviours was reduced.

Surgically-sterilised adult male kangaroos did not show a significant difference in agonistic behaviours during the post-treatment period of observation, neither was there any difference between these groups when comparing pre- and post-treatment observations. This may be due to the relatively short time between surgical procedures and the last set of observations, and persistence of significant levels of testosterone in castrated males. This finding is similar to the results of a study of rock hyrax [24], in which adult males given the orchidectomy procedure still displayed agonistic behaviours when approached by other males, but they were never seen to initiate them. Such behavioural inertia is to be expected given the significant time and learning required for the development of the behaviour. We expect that longer-term observations of our population of kangaroos may show a decrease in initiated agonistic behaviours in castrated male kangaroos, although our current (short-term) data do not demonstrate this.

In contrast to our observations, other studies [25,26] suggest that the display of sexual behaviours is infrequent in sub-adult male eastern grey kangaroos and that only dominant males will 'follow and sniff' the females. We observed a decrease in the sexual behaviours of surgically sterilised sub-adult males in the post-treatment period, when compared with the control (pre-treatment) period. The reason is unclear, but it may be a function of the relatively short period of observation post-treatment or low sampling effort. In the adult males given the orchidectomy procedure, sexual behaviours decreased significantly during the post-treatment observation period, and were almost completely absent by the end of the observation period. The plasma levels of testosterone in the male eastern grey kangaroos following this procedure have not been reported in the literature, although it decreases after just 5 days in tammar wallabies (*M. Eugenii*) [27].

Staker [28] found that macropodid males post-vasectomy did not have decreased agonistic behaviours, which is consistent with the fact that vasectomy does not significantly alter the level of circulating androgens in the body. This is consistent with our observations and those of Bolitho *et al.* [29], who reported similar results in male eastern grey kangaroos given a vasectomy.

In the females, the longer time spent walking may indicate a less cohesive social group, reflecting reduced sexual activity in both males and females. The need for an effective perimeter fence is evident, particularly if there is a resident population outside the target population, as in this study. In the females there was also less time spent scanning, possibly for potential mates, and less time self-grooming, perhaps reflecting less tension in the group as a result of reduced sexual activity. These changes were not observed in previous research using deslorelin in kangaroos [30].

Our study targeted the entire population on the golf course, and approximately 90% of animals were actually treated. This appeared effective in controlling population for several years. If a smaller proportion had been treated, or there had been greater incursion into the course for example as a result of a drought, the duration of reproductive control would diminish.

5. Conclusions

Population management plans involving non-lethal reproductive manipulation are increasingly required to manage landlocked wildlife populations. The development and assessment of effective and humane management techniques are essential if wildlife managers are to appropriately respond to community expectations for compassionate and ethical solutions. Our study demonstrates that although medium-scale kangaroo reproductive management programs are, or can be, effective and achievable, there are nevertheless significant risks to animal welfare that must be mitigated if such programs are to be utilised widely. Key issues affecting animal welfare are generally associated with induction of, and recovery from anaesthesia, during which time kangaroos are susceptible to misadventure and injury. These risks can be mitigated to some degree by minimisation of disturbance and rapid induction of anaesthesia, appropriate confinement during recovery, use of well-trained and experienced personnel, and avoiding darting during warmer months. In spite of the best preparation and precautions we suggest that mortality rates in kangaroos of 5–10% may be expected until better anaesthetic regimes for field darting and chemical restraint become available.

Acknowledgements and Approvals

We acknowledge, with thanks, the assistance of the staff and management of "The Pines Golf Course", Sanctuary Cove, the generous support of volunteers from Wildcare Australia, and staff and volunteers of Australia Zoo, Wildlife Warriors Worldwide Ltd.

Permission to access the site was provided by the management of the golf course. The eastern grey kangaroo is protected under the Queensland *Nature Conservation Act 1992*. Under the provisions of this Act a Damage Mitigation Permit (WIMP04453007) for the reproductive management program itself and a Scientific Purposes Permit (WISP04452507) for the behavioural observations during and after the management interventions were acquired. Animal experimentation ethics approval (SAS/030/07) was provided by the University of Queensland Animal Ethics Committee. All veterinary procedures were conducted by registered veterinary surgeons with wildlife expertise.

References

1. Archer, M.; Grigg, G.; Flannery, T. *The Kangaroo*; Kevin Weldon: McMahons Points, NSW, Australia, 1985.
2. Dawson, T.J. *Kangaroos, Biology of the Largest Marsupials*; University of New South Wales Press Ltd.: Sydney, Australia, 1995.

3. Tribe, A. Managing Kangaroos as a Sustainable Resource. In Proceedings of Annual Conference of the Australian Veterinary Association, Sydney, Australia, 12–17 May 1991; p. 66.

4. Adderton Herbert, C. Long acting contraceptives: A new tool to manage overabundant kangaroo populations in nature reserves and urban areas. *Aust. Mammal.* **2004**, *26*, 67–74.

5. Herbert, C.A.; Trigg, T.E.; Cooper, D.W. Fertility control in female eastern grey kangaroos using the GnRH agonist deslorelin. 1. Effects on reproduction. *Wildl. Res.* **2006**, *33*, 41–46.

6. Coulson, G.; Nave, C.D.; Shaw, D.; Renfree, M.B. Long-term efficacy of levonorgestrel implants for fertility control of eastern grey kangaroos (*Macropus giganteus*). *Wildl. Res.* **2008**, *35*, 520–524.

7. Kitchener, A.L.; Harman, A.; Kay, D.J.; McCartney, C.A.; Mate, K.E.; Rodger, J.C. Immunocontraception of eastern grey kangaroos (*Macropus giganteus*) with recombinant brushtail possum (*Trichosurus vulpecula*) ZP3 protein. *J. Rep. Immunol.* **2009**, *79*, 156–162.

8. Nave, C.D.; Coulson, G.; Poiani, A.; Shaw, G.; Renfree, M.B. Fertility control in the eastern grey kangaroo using levonorgestrel implants. *J. Wildl. Manag.* **2002**, *66*, 470–477.

9. Brooks, R.P.; Fleming, M.W.; Kennelly, J.J. Beaver. Colony response to fertility control: evaluating a concept. *J. Wildl. Manag.* **1980**, *44*, 568–575.

10. Davidson, J.M. Characteristics of sex behaviour in male rats following castration. *Anim. Behav.* **1966**, *14*, 266–272.

11. Ramsey, D. Effects of fertility control on behavior and disease transmission in brushtail Possums , *J. Wildl. Manag.*, **2007**, *71*, 109–116.

12. Zamaratskaia, G.; Rydhmer, L.; Andersson, H.K.; Chen, G.; Lowagie, S.; Andersson, K.; Lundstrom, K. Long-term effect of vaccination against gonadotropin-releasing hormone, using Improvac (TM), on hormonal profile and behaviour of male pigs. *Anim. Rep. Sci.* **2008**, *108*, 37–48.

13. Asquith, K.L.; Kitchener, A.L.; Kaya, D.J. Immunisation of the male tammar wallaby *(Macropus eugenii)* with spermatozoa elicits epididymal antigen-specific antibody secretion and compromised fertilisation rate *J. Rep. Immunol.* **2006**, *69*, 127–147.

14. Kitchener, A.L.; Edds, L.M.; Molinia, F.C.; Kay, D.J. Porcine Zonae Pellucidae Immunization of Tammar Wallabies (*Macropus eugenii*): Fertility and Immune Responses. *Reprod. Fertil. Dev.* **2002**, *14*, 215–223.

15. Coulson, G. Management of overabundant macropods—Are there conservation benefits? In *Managing Marsupial Abundance for Conservation Benefits*; Austin, A., Ed.; Cooperative Research Centre for the Conservation and Management of Marsupials: Sydney, Australia, 1998.

16. Vogelnest, L.; Portas, T. Macropods. In *Medicine of Australian Mammals*; Vogelnest, L., Woods, R., Eds.; CSIRO Publishing: Collingwood, Australia, 2008; pp. 133–225.

17. Coulson, G. Repertoires of social behaviour in captive and free-ranging grey kangaroos, Macropus giganteus and Macropus fuliginosus (Marsupialia: Macropodidae). *J. Zool.* **1997**, *242*, 119–130.

18. Coulson, G. Repertoires of social behaviour in the Macropodoidea. In *Kangaroos, Wallabies and Rat-Kangaroos*; Grigg, G.C., Jarman, P.J., Hume, I.D., Eds.; Surrey Beatty & Sons: Sydney, Australia, 1989; pp. 457–473.

19. Mcdonald, I. University of Queensland, Gatton, Australia. Personal observation, 2008.

20. Vogelnest, L. Chemical Restraint of Australian Native Fauna. In *Wildlife in Australia: Healthcare and Management*; Proceedings 327; Post Graduate Foundation in Veterinary Science, University of Sydney: Sydney, Australia, 1999; pp. 149–187.

21. Arnold, G.W.; Steven, D.; Weeldenburg, J.; Brown, O.E. The use of alpha-chloralose for the repeated capture of western grey kangaroos, *Macropus-fuliginosus*. *Austr. Wildl. Res.* **1986**, *13*, 527–533.

22. Mauthe von Degerfeld, M. Personal experiences in the use of Zoletil for anaesthesia of the red necked wallaby (*Macropus rufogriseus*). *Vet. Res. Comm.* **2005**, *29*, 297–300.

23. Pitt, J.; Lariviere, S.; Messier, F. Efficacy of Zoletil for field immobilization of raccoons. *Wildl. Soc. Bull.* **2006**, *34*, 1045–1048.

24. Manharth, A.; Harris-Gerber, L. Surgical castration and the effect on aggression in rock hyrax (*Procavia capensis). J. Zoo Wildl. Med.* **2002**, *33*, 80–82.

25. Ganslosser, U. Agonistic behavior in Macropodoids—A Review. In *Kangaroos, Wallabies and Rat Kangaroos*; Grigg, G., Jarman, P., Hume, I., Eds.; Surrey, Beatty and Sons: Sydney, Australia, 1989; Volume 2.

26. Hohn, M.; Kronschnabel, M.; Gansloßer, U. Similarities and differences in activites and agonistic behavior of male eastern grey kangaroos (*Macropus giganteus*) in captivity and the wild. *Zoo Biol.* **2000**, *19*, 529–539.

27. Catling, P.C.; Sutherland, R.L. Effect of gonadectomy, season and the presence of female tammar wallabies (*Macropus Eugenii*) on concentration of testosterone, luteinizing hormone and follicle stimulating hormone in the plasma of male tammar wallabies. *J. Endocrinol.* **1980**, *86*, 25–33.

28. Staker, L. *The Complete Guide to the Care of Macropods: A Comprehensive Guide to the Handrearing, Rehabilitation and Captive Management of Kangaroo Species*; Matilda Publishing: Townsville, Australia, 2006.

29. Bolitho, E.; Coulson, G.; Bricknell, S. Body Size, Dominance and Mating Success in Grey Kangaroos. In Proceedings of the 6th International Behaviour Ecology Congress, Canberra, Australia, 29 September–4 October 1996.

30. Woodward, R.; Herbertstein, M.E.; Herbert, C.A. Fertility control in female eastern grey kangaroos using the GnRH agonist deslorelin. 2. Effects on behaviour. *Wildlife Res.* **2006**, *33*, 47–55.

Permissions

All chapters in this book were first published in Animals, by MDPI; hereby published with permission under the Creative Commons Attribution License or equivalent. Every chapter published in this book has been scrutinized by our experts. Their significance has been extensively debated. The topics covered herein carry significant findings which will fuel the growth of the discipline. They may even be implemented as practical applications or may be referred to as a beginning point for another development.

The contributors of this book come from diverse backgrounds, making this book a truly international effort. This book will bring forth new frontiers with its revolutionizing research information and detailed analysis of the nascent developments around the world.

We would like to thank all the contributing authors for lending their expertise to make the book truly unique. They have played a crucial role in the development of this book. Without their invaluable contributions this book wouldn't have been possible. They have made vital efforts to compile up to date information on the varied aspects of this subject to make this book a valuable addition to the collection of many professionals and students.

This book was conceptualized with the vision of imparting up-to-date information and advanced data in this field. To ensure the same, a matchless editorial board was set up. Every individual on the board went through rigorous rounds of assessment to prove their worth. After which they invested a large part of their time researching and compiling the most relevant data for our readers.

The editorial board has been involved in producing this book since its inception. They have spent rigorous hours researching and exploring the diverse topics which have resulted in the successful publishing of this book. They have passed on their knowledge of decades through this book. To expedite this challenging task, the publisher supported the team at every step. A small team of assistant editors was also appointed to further simplify the editing procedure and attain best results for the readers.

Apart from the editorial board, the designing team has also invested a significant amount of their time in understanding the subject and creating the most relevant covers. They scrutinized every image to scout for the most suitable representation of the subject and create an appropriate cover for the book.

The publishing team has been an ardent support to the editorial, designing and production team. Their endless efforts to recruit the best for this project, has resulted in the accomplishment of this book. They are a veteran in the field of academics and their pool of knowledge is as vast as their experience in printing. Their expertise and guidance has proved useful at every step. Their uncompromising quality standards have made this book an exceptional effort. Their encouragement from time to time has been an inspiration for everyone.

The publisher and the editorial board hope that this book will prove to be a valuable piece of knowledge for researchers, students, practitioners and scholars across the globe.

List of Contributors

Birte Stock
Department of Biomedicine, University of Basel, Pestalozzistrasse 20, 4056 Basel, Switzerland

Daniel Haag-Wackernagel
Department of Biomedicine, University of Basel, Pestalozzistrasse 20, 4056 Basel, Switzerland

Jessica P. Hekman
Department of Animal Sciences, University of Illinois at Urbana-Champaign, 1207 West Gregory Drive, Urbana, IL 61801, USA

Alicia Z. Karas
Department of Clinical Sciences, Cummings School of Veterinary Medicine, Tufts University, 200 Westboro Road, North Grafton, MA 01536, USA

Claire R. Sharp
Department of Clinical Sciences, Cummings School of Veterinary Medicine, Tufts University, 200 Westboro Road, North Grafton, MA 01536, USA

Paul Koene
Department of Animal Welfare, Wageningen UR Livestock Research, P.O. Box 65, 8200 AB Lelystad, The Netherlands

Bert Ipema
Department of Farm Systems, Wageningen UR Livestock Research, P.O. Box 65, 8200 AB Lelystad, The Netherlands

Monique Bestman
Louis Bolk Institute, Hoofdstraat 24, 3972 LA, Driebergen, The Netherlands

Jan-Paul Wagenaar
Louis Bolk Institute, Hoofdstraat 24, 3972 LA, Driebergen, The Netherlands

Christelle Tobie
SPF Diana, ZA du Gohélis, Elven 56250, France

Franck Péron
SPF Diana, ZA du Gohélis, Elven 56250, France

Claire Larose
SPF Diana, ZA du Gohélis, Elven 56250, France

Andrew Knight
Ross University School of Veterinary Medicine, P.O. Box 334, Basseterre, St Kitts, West Indies

Ana Raquel Martins
Faculty of Sciences, University of Porto, Rua do Campo Alegre S/N, 4169-007 Porto, Portugal

Nuno Henrique Franco
IBMC — Instituto de Biologia Molecular e Celular, University of Porto, Rua do Campo Alegre 823, 4150-180 Porto, Portugal

Kadri Koppel
Sensory Analysis Center, Department of Human Nutrition, Kansas State University, 1310 Research Park Drive, Manhattan, KS 66502, USA

Mariana Monti
Department of Veterinary Clinic and Surgery, College of Agricultural and Veterinarian Sciences, Sao Paulo State University (UNESP), Via de Acesso Prof. Paulo Donato Castellane, s/n, Jaboticabal, SP 14.884-900, Brazil

Michael Gibson
Department of Grain Science and Industry, Kansas State University, Manhattan, KS 66506, USA

Sajid Alavi
Department of Grain Science and Industry, Kansas State University, Manhattan, KS 66506, USA

Brizio Di Donfrancesco
Sensory Analysis Center, Department of Human Nutrition, Kansas State University, 1310 Research Park Drive, Manhattan, KS 66502, USA

Aulus Cavalieri Carciofi
Department of Veterinary Clinic and Surgery, College of Agricultural and Veterinarian Sciences, Sao Paulo State University (UNESP), Via de Acesso Prof. Paulo Donato Castellane, s/n, Jaboticabal, SP 14.884-900, Brazil

Andrew Tribe
School of Agriculture and Food Sciences, University of Queensland, Gatton, Queensland 4343, Australia
Centre for Animal Welfare and Ethics, University of Queensland, Gatton, Queensland 4343, Australia

Jon Hanger
Endeavour Veterinary Ecology Pty Ltd, Toorbul, Queensland 4510, Australia

Ian J. McDonald
School of Agriculture and Food Sciences, University of Queensland, Gatton, Queensland 4343, Australia

Jo Loader
Endeavour Veterinary Ecology Pty Ltd, Toorbul, Queensland 4510, Australia

Ben J. Nottidge
GreenLeaf Ecology, Mooloolah, Queensland 4553, Australia

Jeff J. McKee
Ecosure, West Burleigh, Queensland 4219, Australia

Clive J. C. Phillips
Centre for Animal Welfare and Ethics, University of Queensland, Gatton, Queensland 4343, Australia

www.ingramcontent.com/pod-product-compliance
Lightning Source LLC
Chambersburg PA
CBHW070245230326
41458CB00099B/5258